Health
and Social Change
in Russia
and Eastern Europe

Health
and Social Change
in Russia
and Eastern Europe

William C. Cockerham

Routledge
New York
London

Preface

The idea for this book had its origin in Vienna at the 1992 meeting of the European Society of Health and Medical Sociology. The Vienna meeting was attended by social scientists and physicians from all over Europe, including several researchers from the former socialist countries. Although it was well known that levels of health and life expectancy were seriously declining in the former Soviet bloc, I found that, both in the presentation of papers and in scholarly dialogue, no one—from either the East or the West—could explain why this situation was occurring.

The lack of an explanation presented itself as an intriguing research question, since rising mortality in the region was obviously one of the most important public health problems in the last decades of the twentieth century. The East and West had taken different routes to modernity and the Eastern approach (the "experiment" in socialism) had disastrous health consequences. Yet this development seemed to be generally overlooked by medical sociologists in the West, especially in the United States; while, in the East, sociology in general and medical sociology in particular were only just regaining strength as academic specialties after being either abolished or relegated to a marginal position in the former Soviet Union and Eastern Europe. Communist regimes did not want sociologists identifying and analyzing social problems when such problems were not supposed to exist; patterns of social stratification were a particularly sensitive issue in societies that were officially "classless." Pointing out that communism was bad for a person's health was not likely to be allowed, either. So given what could be considered a lack of familiarity with the region on the part of most Western social scientists, and the early state of development of free and uncensored medical sociology in the East, it was clear that collaboration between Eastern and Western researchers was the best way to find answers to questions concerning one of the most significant health problems of the late twentieth century: Why

Finland; Stoyanka Popova, Ph.D., Department of Social Medicine and Biostatistics, Medical University, Varna, Bulgaria; Alfred Rutten, Ph.D., Institute of Sports Science, University of Chemnitz, Germany; Stefan L. Rywik, M.D., Ph.D., Director for Research Coordination, National Institute for Cardiology, Warsaw, Poland; and the late Voytek Zubek, Ph.D., Department of Government and Public Service, University of Alabama at Birmingham.

Also I wish to express my appreciation to those persons who helped in the production of this book at the University of Alabama at Birmingham, namely my doctoral student research assistant Christine Snead; and Tenannt McWilliams, Ph.D., Dean, School of Social and Behavioral Sciences, for his unwavering support. I would also like to thank my wife Cynthia and my children Laura, Sean, and Scott for their understanding during this project, and my son Geoffrey, who accompanied me on trips to Hungary, Romania, Poland, and Russia. Finally, I wish to acknowledge the able assistance of Heidi Freund, Liana Fredley, and their associates at Routledge, for their role in making this book a reality.

William C. Cockerham
Birmingham, Alabama

Chapter 1

Introduction

One of the most significant developments in world health in the late twentieth century is the decline in life expectancy in the former Soviet Union and Eastern Europe. This situation is without precedent in modern history. Nowhere else has health worsened so seriously in peacetime among industrialized nations. Ironically, these countries sponsored a communist ideology of socioeconomic equality that theoretically should have promoted health for all. However, the reverse occurred, and life expectancy for many people has been declining for over three decades. This is a surprising development. The likelihood that an entire group of industrialized societies under a stable administrative system would experience such a prolonged deterioration in public health was completely unexpected (Eberstadt 1994:217). Not only is this circumstance a health disaster for the individuals and societies involved, but it also represents an intriguing puzzle to be solved since a full explanation about why this happened has not been forthcoming (Eberstadt 1994; Makara 1994).

The purpose of this book is to solve that puzzle by providing an explanation for the rise of adult mortality in the former socialist countries. Although there are accounts identifying individual risk factors like alcohol abuse, smoking, and poor nutrition as major reasons for the downturn in life expectancy, it will be argued that these factors have their origins in the social conditions and behavioral patterns prevalent in society at large. To claim that alcohol, smoking, or poor eating habits are responsible for the large number of premature deaths does not explain why so many people in the former Soviet-bloc nations drank alcohol, smoked, or consumed less nutritious food to the extent that they significantly shortened their lives. As which workers realize their common oppression, unite, and rise to destroy the prevailing capitalist system.

Marx and his associate Friedrich Engels ([1846]1973:60) emphasized the importance of revolution for changing society by arguing that "the revolution is necessary, therefore, not only because the *ruling* class cannot be overthrown in any other way, but also because the class *overthrowing* it can, only in a revolution, succeed in ridding itself of all the muck of ages and become fitted to found society anew." The alteration of society on a mass scale was therefore possible only through revolution, and it was the historical role of industrial workers to lead the way. Once this occurred and private ownership of the means of production was replaced by collective or state control of the economic system, it would be possible to provide equity in income and living standards to the population at large. "From its origins," observes American political scientist Ronald Suny (1998:xiv), "socialism had the goal of broadening the power of ordinary people, that is, of extending as far as possible the limits of democracy, not only in the realm of politics (which was the goal of democratic radicals and leftist liberals) but in the economy as well." The most unique feature of the socialist economy was the elimination of private property and the institutionalization of collective (usually state) ownership; other characteristics include the restriction of markets, central planning of production, and the intervening role of the state in redistributing goods and services where required (Szelényi, Beckett, and King 1994).

Marx insisted that by abolishing the private ownership of property society would free itself of class antagonisms and begin the transition to a truly classless social structure. Just how this utopia was to be achieved was never fully articulated. There is no hint in Marx's writings about how the transition would take place from the first stage of state ownership of property to the higher stage of full communism marking the establishment of a classless social system. The notion of a classless society, however, remained the ideal end state of socialism. Yet this circumstance never became a reality, nor did socialist states emerge in the West as a result of revolution. Instead, free-market capitalism began producing higher standards of living, which workers, assisted by labor unions, came to share through improved wages, better housing, pensions, and health care plans. State-sponsored welfare programs for the needy and unemployed also came into existence.

It was in the Russian Empire, the largest and most industrially underdeveloped European state, that Marxist doctrine was to have its first success in inducing a revolution. Why Russia? The answer, according to Figes (1996), is that Marxism provided a "scientific doctrine" of social change and did so in the context of a European vision that Russian radicals found attractive. Also important was the sense of optimism and certainty that accompanied Marxism. "It showed," states Figes (1996:140), "that progress lay in industry, that there was meaning in the chaos of history, and that through the working class, through the conscious striving of humanity, socialism would become the end of history."

The Soviet Union

The 1917 Revolution, which toppled the czar and his government, and the subsequent takeover by Vladimir Lenin and the communists made the socialist experiment possible. Based on Marx's vision of socialism, the working class was to control the production of wealth and the future social order was to be founded on the abolition of unearned social privilege, the secularization of society, and the empowerment of working people to run the country (Suny 1998). Equality in access to education and health care, and guaranteed employment were also planned. The Russian Empire was renamed the Soviet Union to reflect its socialist character. And its former class system was destroyed—beginning with the murder of the czar and his immediate family. The nobility had their property confiscated by the state and either fled abroad, were killed or imprisoned, or managed to survive in greatly reduced circumstances. Wealthy landowners, industrialists, and merchants, along with the middle class and affluent peasants, were also purged, and the new Soviet society was reconstituted through upward social mobility from the ranks of workers and peasants.

Tens of thousands of people were killed when Lenin unleashed a terrorist campaign against his foes. But Joseph Stalin, Lenin's successor from 1924 to 1953, went much further, with mass executions, starvation, purges of communists and noncommunists alike, and exile to labor camps where underfed prisoners toiled on construction projects under appalling living conditions. By 1939, the Gulag—the Soviet system of concentration camps—was the largest employer in Europe; altogether, it is estimated that at least 50 million people were victims of Stalin's oppression (Davies 1996). In addition to the vast number of people killed, families destroyed, and lives ruined, Stalin subjected the country to an intense process of industrialization, urbanization, and collectivization of agriculture. There was no empowerment of the people, neither in the Soviet Union nor in the states of Eastern Europe, which were acquired after World War II. The people were never allowed to control the economy they theoretically owned. According to Suny (1998:237):

> Stalin's command economy was hierarchical, with those above issuing orders and expecting obedience from those below. The top officials in Moscow made all the major and many minor decisions concerning industrialization throughout the vast country. Industry was one huge state enterprise with corporate headquarters in the Kremlin. One of Stalin's innovations in Marxist theory was to declare that the state would become stronger before it would disappear altogether: "The higher development of state power in order to prepare conditions for the withering away of state power—this is the Marxist formula."

It is accurate to say that the Soviet Union's socialist experiment was modeled more after Stalin's interpretation of Marx than Lenin's (Davies 1996). American journalist Fred Coleman (1996:13) notes that, in the end, Stalinism was the defining factor in all 74 years of Soviet rule; it was Stalin who became the architect of every major feature of the Soviet system from the command economy to police state repression to the military buildup. Stalin created the superpower that absorbed Eastern Europe into its sphere of domination and developed the capacity for nuclear war. All control was centralized in the Communist Party and the Party answered to Stalin. Once the Party undertook the reconstruction of society, American foreign policy analyst Zbigniew Brzezinski (1989:32) notes, the power of the state had to grow, and it did so to the point of becoming a police state stifling social creativity, suppressing intellectual innovation, and creating a system of hierarchical privilege—all subject to centralized political control. Stalin died in 1953, and many of his crimes were repudiated by his immediate successor, Nikita Khrushchev, who stayed in office until 1964. But the dictatorial structure of government was maintained and major efforts at democratization were not forthcoming until Mikhail Gorbachev assumed power in 1985.

The class system that evolved under Stalin also persisted. The greatest changes were the emergence of a huge working class as the largest component of the Soviet class structure, a corresponding reduction in the rural peasant group, and the installment of *nomenklatura*—the Communist Party elite—at the top of society. This was no classless society. Members of the *nomenklatura* had special privileges with respect to consumer goods and services, housing, health care, vacations, travel abroad, and schools.

At the other end of the social scale, those at the bottom of society—the peasants—had historically been disadvantaged, and this remained true of the population who stayed at this level of the social strata in Soviet times.

One of the better descriptions of Soviet society before its collapse is provided by British historian Norman Davies (1996:1095–6):

> Soviet society, officially classless, was dominated by a growing gulf between the Party elite and the rest of the population. Once the Purges stopped, the members of the *nomenklatura* were able to entrench their position, to purloin state property for their own use, to grow rich and powerful from patronage. The higher echelons were allocated luxury flats and dachas, expensive limousines, exclusive access to closed stores, Western currency, and foreign travel. . . . The collectivized peasants, in contrast, suffered deprivation worse than that of the serfs. Until the 1970s they possessed neither social security benefits nor personal identity papers. The industrial workers were told that they had inherited the earth; they toiled in expectation of the improved housing, wages, and safety which never materialized. The intelligentsia—which in the official definition represented a professional stratum of "brain workers"—enjoyed high prestige but low incomes. Despite the fact that several professions, such as medical doctors, were predominantly females, Soviet women received little relief from conditions that their sisters in the West would not have tolerated. . . . "Developed socialism" was, by European standards, very undeveloped.

Not only socially and politically but also economically the Stalinist system remained in place with its characteristic emphasis upon central planning from Moscow, heavy industry, and the production of weapons. Following World War II, the Soviet Union had become a military superpower and pitted itself in a cold war, along with the Warsaw Pact countries, against the West led by the other superpower, the United States. As Davies points out, the Soviet Union was producing guns, tanks, rockets, and military aircraft in large quantities. But it could not support the needs of its civilian population much beyond state subsidies for food and housing. These guaranteed a subsistence standard of living. Food was produced, but much of it could not be delivered to family kitchens because of poor distribution and transportation systems; few consumer goods were available and poor quality was typical of those sold in the marketplace; outmoded heavy industries continued to turn out steel and iron, largely for the military; and the country's exports were generally limited to armaments, oil, gas, and gold. "By the early 1980s," states Davies (1996:1097), "the combination of uncontrolled military spending and the diminishing returns of domestic performance spelled the onset of system crisis requiring urgent treatment."

Shkolnikov, Meslé, and Vallin 1996a, 1996b). These data do not disguise mortality from cholera, plague, suicide, homicide, and job-related accidents which occurred for political reasons in official publications during the Soviet period (Leon et al. 1997). As Russian demographer Vladimir Shkolnikov and his French colleagues (Shkolnikov et al. 1996a:133) describe the situation:

> In order to maintain correct totals for all causes, death from these concealed causes were included with ill-defined causes. They were, however, tabulated secretly in a special "secret" table which we were finally able to consult for the years 1963–87. Such secrecy is not difficult to understand: in 1970, for instance, the standardized death rate by homicide was almost eight times as high as the European average. The authorities preferred to keep information of this kind, considered politically dangerous, out of reach of observers within and without the Soviet Union.

Deaths from heart disease, however, were not disguised; rather, Soviet policy between 1974 and 1987 was to not publish the information because it was unfavorable. Shkolnikov et al. explain that it was not until 1988 that *perestroika* (restructuring) and *glasnost* (openness) began a new era in Soviet statistics when cause-of-death data were made available by Goskomstat and published systematically. In order to verify the quality of cause-of-death registration data, Shkolnikov et al. reviewed three large-scale surveys conducted in different time periods and in different locales in the Soviet Union. These surveys had been carried out in the early 1960s, 1979, and 1981–82 to check the validity and reliability of mortality data by matching the cause of death entered on death certificates with the "real" diagnosis from medical files and autopsy reports and the coded cause of death. "An interesting feature of the results," state Shkolnikov et al. (1996a:137), "is that they do not support the widespread opinion that cardiovascular mortality has been overestimated." Though some errors were found for individual diseases within the cardiovascular category (i.e., hypertension, rheumatic heart disease, ischemic heart disease, stroke), Shkolnikov and his associates determined that they tended to offset one another and the total error for cardiovascular mortality was small. One survey showed an overregistration of 2%, and the other two surveys showed an underregistration of 2 to 3%. "Thus," conclude Shkolnikov et al. (1996a:137), "the unfavorable trend in cardiovascular mortality in Russia reflects a real deterioration rather than any increasing overestimation."

Virtually all sources maintain that circulatory diseases (ischemic heart disease, stroke, and hypertension) and trauma (accidents, homicide, suicide, and poisonings) dominate the former Soviet bloc's mortality pattern (cf. Cockerham 1997; Eberstadt 1994; Haub 1994; Kaasik, Hörte, and Andersson 1996; Marmot 1996; Marrée and Groenewegen 1997; Notzon et al. 1998; Shkolnikov 1995, 1996; Shkolnikov et al. 1996a, 1996b; Shkolnikov and Nemtsov 1994; Tulchinsky and Varavikova 1996). While it is possible that there were circumstances in which heart disease may have been somewhat overdiagnosed, an upsurge in heart disease appears to be the leading cause of premature death in the former Soviet Union and Eastern Europe (Eberstadt 1994; Haub 1994; Józan 1996a; Marmot 1996) and will be regarded as such in this book. There is too much evidence in support of this conclusion.

SOCIAL CAUSES OF THE RISE IN ADULT MORTALITY

The first question that must be answered is whether or not a social basis exists for this decline in life expectancy. Secondly, if there is a social basis, what is it? Evidence that the downturn primarily resulted from social rather than biomedical causes is supported by the relationship of the rise in mortality with: (1) the sociodemographic characteristics of the people most affected, (2) infectious diseases and genetics, (3) socialist medical care, and (4) environmental pollution.

Sociodemographic Characteristics

It is important to note that the rise in mortality was not universal; rather, there were distinct differences in gender, age, urban/rural locale, education, and region. The people most affected in the former Soviet Union were middle-aged males, with those employed in manual occupations appearing to be the most susceptible (Godek 1995; Haub 1994; Knaus 1981; Mezentseva and Rimachevskaya 1992; Shkolnikov 1995; Tulchinsky and Varavikova 1996). Other data show a similar pattern in Bulgaria (Carlson and Tsvetarsky 1992; Minev, Dermendjieva, and Mileva 1990), the Czech Republic (Carlson and Rychtaříková 1996; Janečková and Hničová 1992; Rychtaříková 1996), East Germany (Häussler, Hempel, and Reschke 1995), Hungary (Carlson 1989; Hungarian Central Statistical Office 1996; Józan 1989, 1996a), Poland

SOURCES: Centrul de Calculsi Statistica Sanitara 1996; *Annual Report of Health and Welfare, 1995–96* (Tokyo: Ministry of Health, 1997); Hungarian Central Statistical Office 1997; State Committee of the Russian Federation on Statistics 1996; *Health United States 1996–97* (Washington, D.C.: U.S. Government Printing Office, 1997); *L'Etat de la France* (Paris: La Decouverte, 1995); National Center for Health System Management 1997; Shkolnikov 1997, *Public Health Statistics Annual, Bulgaria 1995* (Sofia: Ministry of Health, 1996); *Statistical Yearbook of the Czech Republic* (Prague: Czech Statistical Office, 1996); *Statistical Yearbook of the German Democratic Republic* (Berlin: Statistical Office of the German Democratic Republic, 1990); *Statistical Yearbook of the Federal Republic of Germany* (Bonn: Federal Office of Statistics, 1995).

Overall, the data in table 1.1 indicate that male longevity in the region has been considerably worse than that of females. The average length of life for men either decreased (Bulgaria, Hungary, Romania, and Russia) or virtually stagnated and was subject to periodic decline (Czechoslovakia, East Germany, and Poland). Other than Russia, life expectancy for women increased, but the increases were well below that of females in the West and Japan. Table 1.1 shows that, for 1965–94, life expectancy for males increased 6.1 years in France and, for 1965–95, 5.7 years in the United States. In Japan, which has the highest life expectancy in the world for both males and females, longevity for men increased 8.7 years between 1965 and 1995. For women, length of life increased 7.1 years in France, 5.2 years in the United States, and 9.9 years in Japan.

Age-specific contributions to the downturn in life expectancy have been concentrated in middle-aged males throughout the period of decline (Field 1995; Knaus 1981; Mezentseva and Rimachevskaya 1992; Shkolnikov 1995). For example, the greatest increase in death rates for Russian men between 1975 and 1993 is found in the 15–64 age-group, with the most pronounced rise occurring at ages 30–34 (Shkolnikov and Nemtsov 1994). By 1991–92, 54% of all age-specific mortality increases for males were associated with 15- to 44-year-olds and 40% with 45- to 64-year-olds. However, for 1993–94, 53% of the increase in death rates for Russian men was due to excess mortality among 45- to 64-year-olds, 34% to 15- to 44-year-olds, and only 13% to males age 65 and over. Excess mortality in adult males may be shifting to late middle-age in Russia, but nevertheless continues to be a middle-age phenomenon (Shkolnikov 1995, 1996).

The same pattern of rising mortality for middle-aged males also occurs in Eastern Europe, as seen in Bulgaria (Carlson and Tsvetarsky 1992), the Czech Republic (Carlson and Rychtaříková 1996), East Germany (Häussler et al. 1995), Hungary (Carlson 1989; Hungarian Central Statistical Office 1997), Poland (Okólski 1993), and Romania (Muresan

1996; Centrul de Calculsi Statistica Sanitara 1996). As British epidemiologist Michael Marmot (1996) observes, 1992 data show that the 35–64 age-group contributes the most (43%) to the difference in life expectancy between the former Soviet-bloc countries and the rest of Europe. "If socioeconomic factors are important in generating this difference," states Marmot (1996:5202), "they must be operating not only through infant mortality, which is usually thought of as an indicator of socioeconomic conditions, but also through an effect on middle age."

Table 1.1 shows that life expectancy for Russian women generally increased from 1965 to 1991, but with the collapse of communism, already poor health conditions worsened and female life expectancy plunged 3.2 years between 1991 and 1995. And like their male counterparts, it is late-middle-aged (45–64 years) women who have contributed the most to the rise in female mortality since 1992 (Shkolnikov 1996). The accelerated mortality for both men and women in Russia in the 1990s is clearly linked to a definitive social event: the disintegration of the Soviet Union.

As for urban-rural differences in Russia, life expectancy has declined in both locales with urban males showing the greatest decrease. In 1979 urban males outlived rural males by 3 years on average (62.3 years versus 59.3 years), but by 1994 urban males showed an advantage of only 0.8 years (57.7 years versus 56.9 years) over rural males (Shkolnikov 1995). Between 1979 and 1994 life expectancy for urban males declined 4.6 years compared to 2.4 years for rural males, which is shrinking the urban-rural difference. This is an unusual development because urban males in Russia have historically lived longer than their rural counterparts. Rural residents have had to cope with less modern living conditions, lesser-trained health care providers, and more primitive health care delivery, transportation, and communication systems. In 1976, Soviet policy makers tried to improve health in rural areas by concentrating medical personnel and facilities in central locations to provide better quality care. Small hospitals of four beds or fewer were closed, and nurse-midwives were removed from small villages. But in isolated areas with bad roads and no telephones, this policy made it more difficult to obtain both routine and emergency health care. However, despite obstacles to health care delivery in the countryside, the greater decline in longevity for males living in urban areas suggests that life in Russian cities has become especially unhealthy for this group.

Data are lacking on social class differences in mortality because under socialism all strata officially had equal social status. Consequently, there is a paucity of research in the former socialist countries detailing the relationship between health and the three major indicators of socioeconomic status—income, education, and occupational prestige. Among the few existing studies, death rates by education in Russia between 1975 and 1994 for males show increases for all educational groups, with the steepest rise among those with the lowest education (Shkolnikov, Adamets, and Deev 1996). Other data from Poland, Hungary, and Slovakia show a similar association of low education with the highest mortality rates (Bejnarowicz 1994; Ginter 1997; Marmot 1996; Wnuk-Lipinski and Illsley 1990). Given the traditional association in stratification studies of low education with manual labor, the higher mortality rates among less educated Russian men suggests that manual workers were at greatest risk for premature death in the former Soviet Union. And there is evidence to indicate that this is indeed the case among industrial and agricultural laborers (Mezentseva and Rimachevskaya 1992). However, the strongest data come from Bulgaria (Carlson and Tsvetarsky 1992), Hungary (Carlson 1989), and Slovakia (Ginter 1997), where it has been well documented that higher mortality is concentrated among manual workers. Existing research therefore suggests that men employed in occupations requiring manual labor were especially prone to premature deaths in the former socialist countries, although middle-aged men in all social strata were affected to varying degrees.

The rise in adult mortality in the former Soviet Union is also related to region. Table 1.2 compares life expectancy at birth in the former Soviet republics between 1979 and 1980 and either 1991, 1992, or 1993 depending on the availability of data. Surprisingly, the most developed republics in the former Soviet Union's European areas have the greatest declines in life expectancy, while those in the Caucasus and Central Asia generally experienced increases in longevity. The exceptions were Armenia in the Caucasus, where life expectancy fell during this period for both males and females, and Uzbekistan in Central Asia, where a steep decline occurred for females. As shown in table 1.2, the greatest decrease in life expectancy for males was in Russia (-2.5 years), followed by Belarus (-2.1), Latvia (-2.0), Estonia (-1.8), Armenia (-1.6), Lithuania (-0.6), and the Ukraine (-0.6). For females, the decline was greatest in Uzbekistan (-3.2 years), with Armenia (-1.3), Belarus (-1.2), Russia (-1.0), Estonia (-0.4), and Latvia (-0.1) also showing declines.

The lowest standard of living among the former Soviet Republics was in Central Asia, with Tajikistan being the most economically disadvantaged (Keep 1995). Yet table 1.2 shows that Tajikistan had the greatest increase in life expectancy from 1979–80 to the early 1990s of any of the former republics for both males (3.9 years) and females (3.3 years). The highest living standards were present in the Baltic states of Estonia, Latvia, and Lithuania, but life expectancy for males fell in each of these republics and declined for females as well in Estonia and Latvia. Like Russia, the Baltic states have followed the same unfavorable trend in life expectancy (Hertrich and Meslé 1997; Kaasik et al. 1996; Krumins 1997).

Table 1.2

Life Expectancy at Birth in the Former Soviet Republics, 1979–1980 and 1991–1993

Country	Male			Female		
	1979–80	1991–93	Change	1979–80	1991–93	Change
Slavic and Moldova						
Belarus	65.9	63.8	-2.1	75.6	74.4	-1.2
Moldova	62.4	63.9	1.5	68.8	71.9	3.1
Russia	61.5	59.0	-2.5	73.0	72.0	-1.0
Ukraine	64.6	64.0	-0.6	74.0	74.0	0.0
Baltic States						
Estonia	64.2	62.4	-1.8	74.2	73.8	-0.4
Latvia	63.6	61.6	-2.0	73.9	73.8	-0.1
Lithuania	65.5	64.9	-0.6	75.4	76.0	0.6
Caucasus						
Armenia	69.5	67.9	-1.6	75.7	74.4	-1.3
Azerbaijan	64.2	66.3	2.1	71.8	74.5	2.4
Georgia	67.1	68.7	1.6	74.8	76.1	1.3
Central Asia						
Kazakhstan	61.6	63.8	2.2	71.9	73.1	1.2
Kyrgyzstan	61.1	64.2	3.1	70.1	72.2	2.1
Tajikistan	63.7	67.6	3.9	68.6	71.9	3.3
Turkmenistan	61.1	62.9	1.8	67.8	69.7	1.9
Uzbekistan	65.9	66.1	0.2	75.6	72.4	-3.2

*Refers to 1991, 1992, or 1993.
SOURCES: Interstate Statistical Committee of the Commonwealth of Independent States 1995; Haub 1994; Kaasik, Hörte, and Andersson 1996; Shkolnikov 1995.

The general pattern of the rise in mortality is therefore centered on middle-aged, urban males in the most developed republics of the former Soviet Union. Low education and manual labor also appear to be important risk factors. Exclusively biomedical causes of morbidity and mortality would not likely be constrained by these social parameters, thereby indicating that the determinants of the downturn in life expectancy are primarily social. This appears to be the case in Eastern Europe as well.

Infectious Diseases and Genetics

Infectious diseases and genetic changes are not the principal causes of the rise in adult mortality. In the former Soviet Union there was a serious diphtheria epidemic in 1991–96 that infected 200,000 people and took about 5,000 lives over a five-year period. A major flu epidemic also erupted in 1995, while rates of tuberculosis, hepatitis, cholera, and typhoid have increased. Poor public sanitation and lack of proper hygiene (i.e., sterilized instruments, rubber gloves) among health care practitioners and in medical facilities, along with falling rates of vaccination against communicable diseases have been responsible for this development (Garrett 1997). The State Committee of the Russian Federation on Statistics (1996) recorded 17,942 deaths from infectious and parasitic diseases in 1990, which rose to 30,499 in 1995. However, these numbers are quite small compared to mortality from heart disease, which killed 915,498 Russians in 1990 and 1,163,511 in 1995. The mortality rate for infectious and parasitic diseases in Russia in 1995 was 20.7 deaths per 100,000 persons (compared to 12.1 in 1990), while the rate for diseases of the circulatory systems was 790.1 per 100,000 (compared to 617.4 in 1990 and down from 837.3 in 1994). There is a particularly significant increase in mortality rates from accidents, poisonings, and injuries, which nearly doubled between 1990 (133.7 deaths per 100,000 persons) and 1995 (236.6 per 100,000). Most poisonings are from alcohol abuse.

In 1995, diseases of the circulatory system caused 53% of all deaths in Russia, followed by accidents, poisonings, and injuries (16%), cancer (14%), diseases of the respiratory system (5%), diseases of the digestive system (3%), infectious and parasitic diseases (1%), and all other diseases (8%). What is causing the rise in mortality is clearly not an infectious disease spreading largely among middle-aged males, but health problems with direct links to social behavior and conditions that affect these males. Heart disease is the leading culprit, and there has been an upsurge in deaths from accidents, poisonings, and injuries not only in Russia, but also in the former Soviet republics and Eastern Europe (Bojan et al. 1993; Haub 1994; Kaasik et al. 1996; Marrée and Groenewegen 1997; Okólski 1993; Shkolnikov 1996; Shkolnikov et al. 1996a).

A genetic explanation for the health crisis does not seem to apply because the limited time period (approximately 30 years) is not long enough for a large-scale genetic change to have occurred (Adler et al. 1994), nor is there any evidence of genetic change. These conditions do not denigrate the importance of genetic contributions to physical and mental well-being generally; yet a case for a genetic role in the health problems of the former Soviet bloc has not been made, nor is it likely to be forthcoming because of lack of evidence. Although genetics may have been important in the early deaths of some people, since heart disease and alcoholism tend to be more prevalent in some families than in others, there does not appear to be any basis for assigning a genetic origin to the region's widespread health woes.

Socialist Medical Care

Inferior medical care does not seem to be the main cause for the rise in mortality, since there is a lack of support for the claim that socialist health care delivery systems, either by design or inadvertently, are responsible for the widespread deaths of so many people. True, there are long-term problems in the hospitals and clinics of the former Soviet Union with shortages in modern equipment, supplies, and drugs, along with impersonal treatment of patients, overcrowding, and poor hygienic standards (Cassileth, Vlassov, and Chapman 1995; Keep 1995; Knaus 1981). And, with the fall of the Soviet state, conditions have worsened. American journalist Laurie Garrett (1997) observed, for example, that the "former health care delivery system—inefficient, expensive, and authoritarian, but widely accessible—has all but collapsed in the wake of a massive funding crisis, and little has been done to replace it." In former Soviet times only 3 to 4% of the nation's gross domestic product (GDP) was spent on health care, while postcommunist spending has dropped to 1 to 2% of the GDP.

The scarcity of resources has led to the development of inequalities with the best hospitals and medical specialists serving elite groups, and with bribes to physicians and other health care workers being paid for good service. The nation's best medical facilities and best-trained health

Environmental Pollution

While extensive environmental pollution has been found in heavily industrialized and mining areas in the former Soviet Union and Eastern Europe, and there is evidence of an increase in respiratory diseases, hepatitis, lead contamination, and low birth weights in these regions (Hertzman 1995; Keep 1995; Potrykowska 1995), the effects of this pollution are not of such a magnitude as to have caused the massive and nationwide decreases in adult life expectancy (Hertzman 1995; Kulin and Skakkeback 1995; Watson 1995; Wilkinson 1996). This does not mean, however, that the former socialist countries are without serious environmental problems. Communist governments featured strict central planning and did have the authority to prevent pollution. But the emphasis was on industrial development and the indiscriminate exploitation of natural resources in furthering that development. Marxist doctrine held that air, land, and water were a "free" resource for society to appropriate; such resources had no intrinsic value until human labor was applied (Keep 1995). Consequently, little was done under communism to protect the natural environment.

The outcome, as Nagorski (1993:184) points out, is considerable pollution from energy-intensive industries with obsolete equipment which consumed natural resources at an incredible rate. Overreliance on poor-quality, smog-producing brown coal and leaded gasoline resulted in excessive levels of lead, arsenic, nitrogen oxide, sulfur, and dust being released into the air: metallurgy and petrochemical industries contaminated the environment with cadmium, beryllium, and petroleum products; and, in agriculture, overuse of pesticides, herbicides, and fertilizers was widespread (Rose and Bloom 1994).

Even though the situation in the former Soviet Union is not well documented, enough information exists to show that air pollution is a serious problem in many areas; several rivers and lakes are polluted; the size of the land-locked Aral Sea has been reduced by 40% because of water diverted for irrigation projects, and the water that remained has three times more salt, which ruined fishing; and Lake Baikal, the largest and oldest natural reservoir of fresh water in the world, has been contaminated by pulp and paper mills (Keep 1995). The nuclear accident at Chernobyl in the Ukraine in April 1986, a result of policy and design faults in the power plant's equipment, caused radiation to render some 25% of the land uninhabitable in neighboring Belarus. Thousands of villages were closed and cattle slaughtered; numerous factories were shut down and people transported to live elsewhere. Specter (1996) found that ten years after the accident some 20 out of 21 agricultural districts in the contaminated area—one of the most fertile in Belarus—produced nothing. "All normal life stopped here," states Specter (1996:4), "simply because there was a strong northerly wind on April 26, 1986."

The "black triangle" of the largely deforested high plateaus where the German, Czech, and Polish borders meet is one of the most polluted areas in Europe. The eastern part of the basin below the Ore Mountains in North Bohemia of the Czech Republic may possibly be the most environmentally damaged in the world (Janečková and Hniličová 1992). Hertzman observes that the physical and chemical environments of this area are uniquely hostile. "Anyone who visits the mining districts of Teplice, Usti nad Labem, Most, Decin, and Chomutov," Hertzman (1995:19) observes, "will witness the incremental effects of decades of open-pit mining nad effluents from a variety of polluting industries with old technology and poor environmental controls." Emissions from home heating combine with industrial emissions to produce high concentrations of sulfur dioxide in the air, especially during temperature inversions. Adult and infant mortality rates in North Bohemia are the highest in the Czech Republic. Across the border in Katowice Province in Polish Silesia, with 2% of Poland's land and 11% of its population, the area's coal-burning furnaces, coking plants, mines, and chemical factories produce between 30 to 40% of the nation's total air pollution. According to Nagorski (1993:183), "the soil is so laced with hazardous substances that growing garden vegetables is considered an act of recklessness." Not surprisingly, Katowice has the highest mortality rates of any Polish province.

The extent of pollution in the former socialist countries would suggest that ecological devastation may indeed be a major factor in rising adult mortality. Yet, as previously stated, this does not seem to be the case. A major problem with the environmental pollution explanation is that the regions with particularly high levels of pollution do not necessarily have the worst health. East Bohemia in the Czech Republic, for instance, has relatively high life expectancy despite poor air quality, while parts of Slovakia with clean air have low life expectancy (Hertzman 1995). North Bohemia has extensive ecological pollution and, as noted, the highest mortality rates, but rates of cancer are not high relative to the rest of the country (Institute of Health Information and Statistics of the Czech Republic 1997). Compared to the city of that women were not suited to work requiring heavy lifting or skilled labor persisted (Suny 1998). Therefore, for men, and less so for women, working-class membership is an important variable.

Since there was not a life-threatening biological phenomenon or communicable disease that preyed largely on middle-aged working-class males in former socialist societies, the key to understanding the rise in mortality is to be found in the social conditions engendered by those societies. This particular group of men found themselves subject to ways of living that promoted unhealthy behavior that led, in turn, to accelerated levels of heart disease, alcohol consumption, accidents, murder/suicide, and other afflictions. And this was the case not only in the former Soviet Union, but in the rest of the Warsaw Pact countries as well. It is apparent that a social basis exists for the decrease in life expectancy. The next step, accordingly, is to identify the major social determinants, which is the focus of the following chapter.

Chapter 2

The Social Determinants of the Decline in Longevity

It is not completely accurate to say that the health crisis in the former Soviet bloc has been brought about by the socialist vision of society; rather, the crisis seems to be one outcome of European socialism's unsuccessful efforts at modernization (Watson 1995). The 1950s and early 1960s were a time of dynamic economic growth in the region, but efforts to overtake the West faltered thereafter and this period also marked the onset of rising mortality from natural causes. A review of this situation suggests that socialist health policy, societal stress, or health lifestyles are the most likely social determinants of the premature mortality. Were the health policies of the communist regimes so ineffective that scores of middle-aged men died early deaths for more than 30 years? Or were the stresses produced by adverse societal conditions—such as a failing and stagnant economy—at fault? Or were unhealthy styles of living associated with communism the major culprit? These questions are examined in chapter 3.

Socialist Health Policy

Health care delivery systems and policies are acts of political philosophy; therefore, social and political values underlie the choices made, institutions formed, and levels of funding provided for health (Light 1986). Prior to the collapse of communism in the former Soviet Union and

Eastern Europe in 1989–91, the health care delivery systems in the region were philosophically guided by Marxist-Leninist programs for reshaping capitalism into socialism. As previously discussed, the ultimate goal of Marxism-Leninism was the establishment of a classless society, featuring an end to class oppression, private property, worker alienation, and economic scarcity (Bell 1991; Zotov 1985). However, Marxist-Leninist ideology pertaining to health was never developed in depth (Deacon 1984; Field 1967; Marx and Engels 1973; Waitzkin 1983, 1989). Friedrich Engels, Karl Marx's collaborator and sponsor, did publish a major treatise in 1845 linking the poor health of the English working class to capitalism, but he never returned to the topic, and health care was not a central concern in Marxist-Leninist ideology (Waitzkin 1983).

The new Soviet state established in the aftermath of the 1917 Revolution nevertheless faced very serious health problems, including large-scale typhus and cholera epidemics and mass starvation. Vladimir Lenin and the communists had inherited a country that was on the verge of collapse. The economy was ruined, a civil war was raging, and epidemics were spreading among a malnourished and impoverished population. The stability of the new regime was so threatened by disease in 1919 that Lenin proclaimed: "Either the louse defeats socialism or socialism defeats the louse" (Barr and Field 1996:307). More out of practical than theoretical necessity, the Fifth All-Russian Congress of Soviets formulated the basic principles of Soviet health policy in 1918. The Congress mandated that health care would be (1) the responsibility of the state, (2) provided without cost to the patient, (3) controlled by a central authority, and (4) allocated priority of care to workers, with (5) an emphasis on preventive care (Cassileth, Vlassov, and Chapman 1995; Light 1986). In the 1920s, the Soviets established a rudimentary nationwide system of public clinics. Because of the critical need for doctors and the shortage of manpower due to industrial and military needs, large numbers of women, especially nurses with working-class and peasant backgrounds, were ordered into medical schools. They were given cram courses, certified as doctors, and sent out to practice medicine. According to American physician William Knaus (1981:83):

> Many [of these women] had no ambitions beyond a weekly paycheck. The Soviet government responded in kind with a low wage scale and a social status for medicine that treated the new physician with no more respect than that given a factory worker. Professionalism was not rewarded nor even encouraged. Medicine became a job and women were the ones chosen to do it.

By 1990, the year before the collapse of the Soviet Union, the Russian Soviet Federated Socialist Republic had one of the highest numbers of doctors per capita in the world (about one physician for every 259 people), and some 76% of doctors were women (Cassileth et al. 1995). The Soviet government provided low wages (about $24 a month, less than what a bus driver would make) and status (the equivalent of a high school teacher) for the great majority of its medical practitioners. There were some elite doctors, however, who served important people and worked in the best hospitals; other leading physicians were employed in government posts and medical schools as administrators, professors, or consultants for policy decisions. These doctors were usually men who received considerably higher salaries than the average practitioner (Field 1994).

However, most doctors were not in the elite category and had relatively low salaries and status. As American physician Barrie Cassileth and his Russian and American colleagues (Cassileth et al. 1995:1570) point out: "Set by the state, the Soviet wage structure placed coal miners and other heavy industrial workers at the top of the scale and service workers such as physicians and teachers at the lowest extreme." In 1987 the average salary for health care providers was 71% of the national average (Mezentseva and Rimachevskaya 1992). The great majority of Soviet doctors were low-priority employees in a vast national system of health financed directly from the budget of the central government.

The Soviet system of health care delivery was formally established in July 1918 when Lenin authorized the Commissariat for Health Protection. The control, administration, and planning of the nation's health services were centralized in this office. A hierarchical system of health delivery facilities was established, known as the Semashko model after its designer N. A. Semashko. Local polyclinics (outpatient clinics) were the initial point of entry for primary and basic specialist care, as well as the source of referrals to higher-level services and hospitals. As shown in figure 2.1, the central government provided a budget to local governments who, in turn, financed the polyclinics and hospitals that furnished the services to meet patient needs. The general public did not have a choice of physicians, but were assigned to a medical practitioner on the basis of residence.

According to Mark Field (1994), the history of early Soviet medicine can be divided into two phases. The first phase, from the Revolution to the late 1920s, was dominated by social hygienists and hard-core Marxists who believed in the literal truth of Marx's vision of communism. This group, Field (1994:185) observes, maintained that "illness and premature mortality were the product of a 'sick' social system (cap-

Figure 2.1

Structure of the Soviet Health Care Delivery System

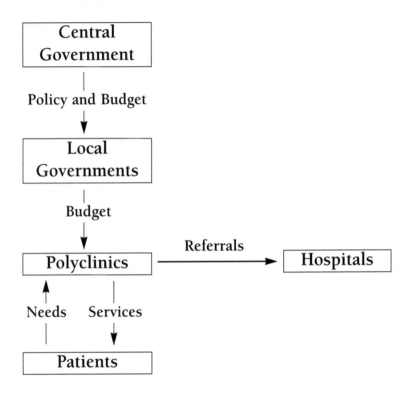

italism) and that the advent of socialism and eventually communism would usher in a new period in human history—one that would be increasingly free of the socially produced ills and evils of the former system." The pathway to a healthy society was through social reform in which pathological conditions engendered by capitalism—namely, poverty, prostitution, alcoholism, drug abuse, and unsafe workplaces—were to be eliminated. The focus of health policy was to be toward prevention rather than medical care. That is, the correction of the social ills that caused people to be unhealthy needed to be the first goal, not the provision of health care. Although consistent with Marxism, this phase was ended by Stalin in the 1930s. As part of his program to force industrialization and collective agriculture, Stalin reoriented Soviet medicine toward keeping people healthy to perform their jobs.

Providing health care to workers with an emphasis on prevention remained the top priority, but medicine was redirected from helping to transform society to supporting economic development and the drive toward modernization. As Field (1994:186) points out, the creation of a reorganized All-Union Commissariat (later Ministry) of Health Protection in 1936 underscored the Soviet commitment to centralization, standardization, and control at the national level that placed medical care and public health directly under the authority of the Party and the state. Physicians were low-wage government employees without any professional power to defend their interests against state control. Professional autonomy was generally limited to decisions about patient care. Medical doctors were, in fact, directly accountable to the state for the health of their patient population and required to keep detailed records; they were judged and remunerated by the medical bureaucracy more by quantitative indicators (numbers of visits and procedures) than the quality of care provided (Remennick and Shtarkshall 1997). "Indices such as volumes of services," states Russian demographer Boris Rozenfeld (1996:163), "were considered sufficient indicators of growing state activity in public health protection and care." As Knaus (1981:352) explains:

> At the same time the collective attitude that was promoted as the basis of the new Soviet state, and that was encouraged in agriculture and industry as one way of coping with regional and national shortages, found its way into medical care. Independent decisions by physicians were discouraged and, as a result, individual responsibility slowly declined. As the years went by dominance of national priorities over the needs of individuals not only changed the character of the doctor-patient relationship in Soviet Russia, it also limited the vision and challenges to which Soviet medicine and Soviet physicians aspired.

The outcome was the establishment of a health care system designed primarily to serve the interests of the state. Thus, the state, not the individual, assumed responsibility for health and provided services as a benefit of communism. According to Rozenfield (1996:164):

> The paternalistic approach manifested itself in the slogan, "The State cares for the health of its citizens," which in many ways defined the very character of medical service organizations across the country, as well as people's attitudes toward this sphere of policy. According to this approach, every person is under the umbrella of the State and its medical facilities, which undertake entire responsibility for his or her health. In this way, a health care system was created which found itself fully dependent on the state and its governing bodies.

Although Soviet primary care doctors had undergone a distinct process of deprofessionalization at the hands of the government, they exercised considerable authority and power over patients (Remennick and Shtarkshall 1997). They were the first line of treatment for ills and discomfort and the source of drug prescriptions, authorization for sick leave, and referrals to hospitals and specialists. To obtain better, more personalized care, patients gave doctors, nurses, and hospital orderlies gifts, services, or monetary payments. Health care personnel, on their part, frequently demanded money for the services they were supposed to provide for free (Barr and Field 1996). This under-the-table income helped offset the low wages of the practitioners, ensured at least a basic level of efficiency, and was a form of barter typical throughout the Soviet economy (Remennick and Shtarkshall 1997). Without these incentives, the average patient had little ability to influence the course of his or her treatment.

When it came to special or individual attention, the Soviet system of medicine was often a failure. As a national program aimed at providing basic services with scarce resources it was a qualified success (Curtis, Petukhova, and Taket 1995; Knaus 1981). Treatment for infectious diseases, immunizations, maternal and child care, and other primary services were widely available (Rowland and Telyukov 1991; Tulchinsky and Varavikova 1996). Although the quality was uneven and services in distant rural areas were provided by physician assistants (*feldshers*) instead of doctors, the Soviets nonetheless established a nationwide health care delivery system providing treatment that was free in theory if not always in fact.

This was a major improvement over the czarist period. In 1897 the Russian Empire was predominately agrarian with 86% of its population living in rural areas; as late as 1928 some four-fifths of all Russians were peasants (Pipes 1995; Suny 1998). Residents of cities and towns might have had access to doctors, but this was rarely the case in the countryside. Some estates of the landed gentry had infirmaries and physicians who could be brought from nearby towns; however, the bulk of the peasant population relied for health care on members of the landowning families, midwives, other peasants with rudimentary paramedical training, folk healers, or simply folk remedies (Roosevelt 1995; Tian-Shanskaia 1993). Nearly half of all Russian peasant children died before the age of five—one of the highest mortality rates recorded anywhere. Most of these deaths were caused by diarrhea and respiratory diseases and only the parents, a midwife, or a village healer would be on hand to help as best they could (Tian-Shanskaia 1993). Not surprisingly, Russia had the highest infant mortality rate in Europe just before World War I; 245 infants per 1,000 died before the age of one compared to 76 per 1,000 in Sweden (Suny 1998). Adult life expectancy was also low, with 1887 figures showing Russians living only 32 years on average; by 1918, longevity had fallen to 30 years in the aftermath of war and rebellion.

The establishment of a geographically homogeneous and centrally planned system providing universal access to professional health care was regarded by the Soviet government as one of its greatest achievements. The initial results were impressive. Between 1928 and 1941, an enormous expansion in numbers of physicians and health facilities took place. Western observers like American physician Henry Sigerist (1947:32) found the early development of the Soviet health care delivery system to be "stupendous." "The chief impression of the visitor in 1938," states Sigerist (1947:32), "was that not only was there more of everything but that more of everything there had been greatly improved." Medical measures, along with some improvements in living standards, were credited with substantially reducing infant mortality and the incidence of many communicable diseases like typhus, cholera, and syphilis.

From the end of World War II until the mid-1960s, health progress in the Soviet Union was rapid, steady, and widespread (Eberstadt 1994; Mezentseva and Rimachevskaya 1990). For example, in the Russian Soviet Federated Socialist Republic life expectancy for males was 40.4 years in 1938 but reached 64 in 1965; for females, life expectancy increased from 46.7 years to 72.1 during that same period. A similar situation occurred in Eastern Europe, where socialist-style health care delivery systems based on the Soviet model had been installed after 1945 (Eberstadt 1994; Okólski 1993). In Hungary, for instance, male life expectancy rose from 54.9 years in 1941 to 67.5 years in 1966—the highest ever recorded (Hungarian Central Statistical Office 1996). Life expectancy for Hungarian females increased from 58.2 years to 72.2 during the same time. A similar pattern existed in Bulgaria, where in 1935–39 life expectancy for males was 51 years; in 1965–67, Bulgarian males lived 68.8 years on average—again, the highest ever recorded in that country (National Center of Health Informatics 1995). For Bulgarian females, life expectancy climbed from 52.6 years in 1935–39 to 72.7 years in 1965–67.

However, in the mid-1960s, life expectancy for males, as discussed in the previous chapter, began a downward trend throughout the Soviet bloc. A review of the literature suggests four major shortcomings in socialist health policy and modes of health care delivery: funding, quality, access, and strategy.

Funding

Health care was not a national priority and was therefore seriously underfunded. In 1989, two years before the Soviet Union collapsed, only 3.4% of the GDP—a percentage lower than in any other industrialized nation—was spent on health care. Turkey (3.9%) and Greece (5.1%), for example, spent larger proportions of their GDP on health that year than the Soviet Union. According to Russian demographers Elena Mezentseva and Natalia Rimachevskaya (1992), health care in the Soviet union was financed on the basis of the "residue principle," that is, from funds left over after providing for the needs of the sectors of the economy given a higher priority: defense, heavy industry, and agriculture.

The Soviet Union was locked into intense political and military competition with the West; its chosen economic system was unprofitable in the face of rising costs, fixed prices, limits on growth, and centralized controls that discouraged innovation (Skidelsky 1995). While the West was moving out of the industrial stage and through a postindustrial era, with the service sector (finance, information, transportation, legal, education, food, insurance, tourism, and other services) becoming the dominant economic activity, the Soviet Union remained mired in an industrial phase. Moreover, computerization placed the Soviets at a distinct disadvantage since their police state controls repressed the creative and uncensored flow of information. Soviet state revenues were falling and could not be restored without reform, yet reform was resisted because the central planning system served the welfare of the *nomenklatura*, the Party, and the state. As Robert Skidelsky (1995:109) comments:

> Shortages and queues for practically everything became universal as wages outstripped consumer-goods production, leaving a "monetary overhang" for bribery and the black economy. Transport, infrastructure, storage and distribution, and social services were neglected. Agriculture stagnated, despite spectacular land-reclamation projects.

In this context, strong financial support for health care delivery was increasingly less likely. The provision of health care by the central government did not produce revenue for the state; quite the contrary, it was a state service draining funds out of the budget. Given its low priority in relation to other state needs, it is not surprising that funding contracted as pressure on the state budget increased. During the Brezhnev era (1964–82), the health care delivery system began to deteriorate. Less and less money was provided and what was available largely went to hospitals, leaving the primary care sector especially impoverished and without basic supplies (Remennick and Shtarkshall 1997). The best estimates are that about 6% of the Soviet Union's GDP was spent on health care in the mid-1960s, but fell to 3% by the time Mikhail Gorbachev took power in 1985 (Field 1994, 1995; Specter 1995). In the new Russian Federation under Boris Yeltsin, health spending dropped to less than 1% of the GDP in 1995 but recovered to 2.2% in 1997.

The funding situation was better in Eastern Europe. Typically these nations followed the Soviet lead in budget priorities, but countries like Hungary and Poland spent slightly more of their GDP on health than the Soviet Union in the 1970s (Deacon 1984). In the late 1980s official health expenditures for Eastern Europe as a whole averaged 5.4% of the region's GDP (Rowland and Telyukov 1991), while the Soviet Union was averaging around 3%. The average in the OECD countries (the West and Japan) at this time was 7.4% of the GDP (Schieber, Poullier, and Greenwald 1994). Thus, the Eastern European countries were at a midpoint between the Soviet Union (low) and the West (high) in health spending. In 1987–89, for example, some 5.2% of the GDP was spent on health in East Germany. In 1989, 5.8% was spent in the former Czechoslovakia, 5.7% in Poland, and 4.6% in Hungary. By way of comparison, Great Britain spent 6% of its GDP on health in 1989, while West Germany spent 8.2 percent, France 8.8 percent, and the United States 11.7%.

Official government statistics, however, actually underestimate the amounts spent on health because of the widespread practice of gifts, services, or bribes paid to health care workers by patients for better service. These "gratuities" probably increased physicians' incomes by 30 to 40% (Marrée and Groenewegen 1997). Nevertheless, even with out-of-pocket payments by patients, it is clear that health services were seriously underfunded by the communists. Since the collapse of communism, health spending has fallen to disastrous levels in Russia (1 to 2%) but risen to 7.3% of the GDP in the Czech Republic in 1993, 7.1% in Hungary in 1993, and 6% in the Slovak Republic in 1994. In Poland, health spending fell to 4.4% of the GDP in 1994, down from 5.3% in 1992 and 4.7% in 1990. Yet Poland is still spending a much higher proportion of its GDP on health than Russia as both nations struggle to develop a market economy. In the meantime, health remains a relatively low priority in former Soviet-bloc policies as socialist-style health care delivery systems remain in place and reflect little or no change from socialist times. Although private fee-for-service care is available to the affluent, few health insurance programs exist, and services generally remain a state responsibility and paid by the central budget.

Quality

Soviet health care was not generally of a high quality in comparison to the West. Although modern facilities and well-trained physicians existed, the great majority of doctors lacked the training of Western physicians and most hospitals were poorly equipped and had inadequate supplies (Cassileth et al. 1995; Curtis et al. 1995; Davis 1989; Keep 1995; Light 1992; Marrée and Groenewegen 1997). As discussed in chapter 1, nearly half of all Soviet hospitals in 1990 lacked hot water, showers, and bathrooms, while 15% were without running water (Cassileth et al. 1995). Many hospitals in other Soviet-bloc countries were in a similar condition (Nagorski 1993). Also, as noted, rural areas were often served by physician assistants in relatively primitive health stations. Soviet medical technology lagged behind that of the West by several years (Makara 1994). Therefore, as American sociologist Donald Light (1992) points out, the widespread availability of competent physicians with the medical supplies needed for their work has been a fundamental problem.

Access

Despite socialist ideology, access to quality health care was inherently unequal in the Soviet system. According to Mezentseva and Rimachevskaya (1992), the existence of social inequality in health care was never described by the government as a problem that needed solving, nor widely recognized as a problem by the general public until only late in the final years of the Soviet regime. What Soviet health policy provided was a universal and equal right to health protection, not an end to socially determined differences in health or in the quality of medical care provided. There was, for example, a complex, stratified arrangement of clinics and hospitals, with separate closed systems for elite groups, such as top government officials, the military, KGB, miners and other industrial workers, and open systems for residents of Moscow, provincial cities, and rural areas.

According to American social scientist Timothy Colton (1995), who studied Moscow's socialist municipal government, when members of the elite were sick, four unmarked polyclinics with a strict order of status were available. First was the original infirmary for this group, followed by (in rank order) the Moscow Clinical Center near Moscow State University and clinics in the Arbat and Presnya areas. These clinics, along with two hospitals, were operated expressly for their exclusive clientele by the Fourth Chief Directorate of the Soviet Ministry of Health. Colton (1995:25) states:

> The carrying capacity of the Fourth Chief Directorate's words and clinics roughly matched the class of the beneficiaries of the Kremlin [district]. In 1990, by which time it had been renamed and some economies were made, the directorate had 23,649 patients on register in Moscow. Care was provided by 19,414 health personnel, with an average annual expenditure of 1,400 rubles per patient—as compared to between 40 and 100 rubles per patient in standard municipal organizations.

Colton adds that the Central Clinical Hospital for the Moscow power elite had the best medical doctors in the country and one of the polyclinics for this group had more than 1,000 personnel for its 190 beds, diagnostic clinic, pool, and tennis courts. A step down the social ladder, the Fourth Directorate of the Russian Soviet Federated Socialist Republic Ministry of Health (for the former Russian Republic, not the Soviet Union) operated three polyclinics and two large hospitals for their charges. The Ministries of Defense and Transportation, the KGB, the Academy of Sciences, and other government agencies and ministries had their own clinics and hospitals. Staffing was considerably more generous than in facilities operated by the city health service, there were fewer patients, and doctors and nurses were paid higher than normal salaries. Some 500,000 Moscow residents or about 18% of the city's population of 8.97 million people in 1989 had access to these special health facilities. They avoided the lines in city clinics that the other 82% of Muscovites contended with when they sought care, while having access to better facilities and doctors.

The Eastern European countries had a similar hierarchy of health care services with those at the top of socialist society utilizing the best care available (Nagorski 1993). For example, as in the former Soviet Union, the East German government established a highly stratified network of health facilities, and large inequities in financial support existed. Altogether, some 14 separate health care systems were maintained, including ones for top party officials and diplomats, police, military, the secret police (STASI), construction workers, uranium miners, transportation workers, other industrial workers, academics, university staffs, victims of fascism, elite athletes, church hospitals, and the public system (Volpp 1991). The latter featured long waiting lines and shortages in medical supplies because of its low priority. Despite the fact that the health field was to be an area in which the superiority of socialism could be demonstrated, health care privileges existed for elite groups (Apelt 1991).

Strategy

The strategy emphasizing prevention was not a complete success. The public health tradition favored by the former socialist states was that of secondary prevention or the early detection of disease; much less attention was given to primary prevention, namely the adoption of healthy lifestyles. So the focus was not on actually preventing the onset of a disease (except through immunization), but on detecting it in its early stages so it could be cured more easily or prevented from becoming more serious. This was a major policy mistake because when heart disease, as a chronic incurable illness, was detected, it was too late. Furthermore, this approach was flawed in its execution. For instance, beginning in the mid-1980s in the former Soviet Union, large-scale public health campaigns featuring mandatory screening of the entire adult population were required of the nationwide system of polyclinics. But the effort was often ineffective because of the heavy workload of doctors, a lack of motivation by the participants, and poor follow-up of detected cases (Remennick and Shtarkshall 1997).

Nevertheless, there were some successes. Until the 1990s, the Soviet approach was generally effective in controlling the major infectious diseases (Tulchinsky and Varavikova 1996). There was also some improvement in infant mortality as previously noted, and in deaths from cancer and respiratory diseases between 1970 and 1986 (Mezentseva and Rimachevskaya 1990, 1992). However, mortality from heart disease rose significantly, with age-standardized death rates from circulatory disease increasing in Russia from 814.3 per 100,000 in 1970 to 1,089.3 in 1993 (Shkolnikov 1996; Shkolnikov and Nemtsov 1994).

Whereas socialist health policy was oriented toward the prevention of infectious diseases, it was ineffective in adjusting to the increased prevalence of heart disease and trauma (accidents, alcohol poisonings, homicide, and suicide) in the former Soviet Union and elsewhere in countries like the former Czechoslovakia and Hungary (Bojan, Hajdu, and Belicza

1991; Makara 1994). This leads to the paradoxical conclusion that the centralized egalitarianism that succeeded in addressing epidemics and contagious disease in the early period of Soviet health care delivery functioned poorly when confronted with chronic illnesses and their causes in the late twentieth century. Thus, the Soviet-style health policy did not cause the increase in mortality in the region but rather was unable to stop the surge in circulatory disease and traumatic episodes. The social stress and lifestyles explanations seem to be more promising lines of inquiry in the search for the leading cause of increased mortality.

SOCIAL STRESS

A social stress explanation maintains that differences in health and life expectancy are based on differing capabilities of the various social classes in buffering the effects of stress. Stress can be defined as a heightened mind-body reaction to stimuli inducing fear or anxiety in the individual. Typically, stress begins with a situation that the individual finds troublesome or burdensome. The fears and anxieties associated with this situation, if prolonged, are capable of producing serious psychological distress and physiological reactions that impair health and a sense of well-being. While much of the research concerning stress focuses on small group interaction or micro-level stressors that affect individuals in their everyday life, macro-level stressors originating in the wider society also promote stress. That is, society can create stressful situations that force people to respond to conditions not of their own choosing. The collapse of communism is a good example of such a situation. Regardless of whether or not the changes associated with this event were seen as positive or negative by the people directly experiencing them, lives changed dramatically as the socialist social system disintegrated.

Although stress affects individuals, a powerful body of research documents the fact that the impact of stress varies according to social class position (Cockerham 1998; Marmot 1996; Marmot, Shipley, and Rose 1984; Marmot et al. 1991; Pearlin 1989). It is also clear that socioeconomic distinctions in mortality and morbidity are found for practically all diseases and occur at every level of a social hierarchy, not just between the upper and lower classes (Adler et al. 1994; Illsley and Baker 1991; Marmot 1996). Therefore, something more than poverty is operative in determining health differences between social classes, since the upper class lives longer than the upper-middle class even though both classes are affluent. Thus, the critical factor in health, according to a social stress explanation, is a person's location in a social hierarchy, with higher socioeconomic status providing less exposure to negative situations and more social, psychological, and economic resources in coping with such events when they occur (Adler et al. 1994)

Building upon previous research, a team of American, British, and Canadian researchers led by Robert Evans, Morris Barer, and Theodore Marmor (1994) identifies stress as the single most important variable in the health of large populations. The basis for this conclusion is largely derived from Michael Marmot's (Marmot et al. 1984, 1991) influential Whitehall studies which document a clear social gradient in life expectancy across ranks of British male civil servants. Drawing also upon a variety of studies of social hierarchies of both humans and primates, Evans (1994) finds that those at the top of a society are less affected by stress and have fewer health problems including heart disease. Greater anxiety, higher-level and more prolonged stress responses, along with poorer overall health and more heart disease are characteristic of those at the bottom. Social factors like self-esteem, self-direction in work, control over one's environment, and sense of social support— all variables that decline in strength as one descends the social ladder— are identified as crucial to buffering and/or coping with stress and its physiological impact on the body.

Evans therefore suggests that the social gradient in life expectancy from high to low is generally caused by differing "microenvironments" (defined as relations at home or work) that facilitate the transfer of strain from stressful life events. The lower a person's social class position, the less able that person is to transfer stress, and the greater the harm to the individual's health. Evans claims that it is this ability to transfer or buffer stress, rather than some mechanical connection to wealth, that ultimately determines the effects of stress on the body. Increasing prosperity and success are also cited by Evans as major sources of self-esteem and empowerment—which reflect positively upon an individual's mental and physical health.

Applying this perspective to macro-level processes, Evans and his colleagues (Evans 1994; Evans and Stoddard 1994; Hertzman, Frank, and Evans 1994) note that as Japan has risen to the top of the economic hierarchy of nations in the twentieth century, Japanese life expectancy has become the highest in the world. Russia and Eastern Europe, in contrast, descended in the same hierarchy and witnessed a corresponding decline in life expectancy. This situation suggests that changes in status can be translated into changes in mortality as societal stress is either reduced or increased.

However, while this conclusion has a certain logical appeal in support of the social gradient thesis, it is not at all clear how the relationship between stress and macro-level social change enhances or lessens the life expectancy of large populations, or particular individuals within those populations. Specific stressors and specific disease outcomes have not been identified, which makes it difficult to prove a precise cause and effect. Furthermore, among the Japanese, Okinawans traditionally have the highest longevity, but also have the lowest per capita incomes in Japan and have been accorded lower social status by Japanese in the home islands (Cockerham, Yamori and Hattori 1998). While it might be argued that Okinawan longevity in relation to socioeconomic status is atypical, the fact remains that they are an exception to any hierarchical theory of human life expectancy.

It is apparent that Russia and Eastern Europe comprise societies experiencing considerable stress as a result of fundamental economic, political, and social changes in the wake of communism's downfall (Keep 1995; Leon and Shkolnikov 1998; Stokes 1993). Yet it is not evident that this macro-level stress is the primary cause of the increased mortality. For example, in the former Soviet Union, Tajikistan was the least affluent republic but showed the greatest increase in life expectancy for both men and women between 1979–80 and 1991–93 (see table 1.2 in chapter 1). Other than Armenia, longevity declined in the republics with the highest levels of economic development, namely, Russia, the Baltic states, Belarus, and the Ukraine. Consider also the case of the Czech Republic, which, like the other communist nations, experienced an increase in male mortality beginning in the mid-1960s. But unlike the others, this trend was reversed in the mid-1980s—prior to the end of Soviet domination and the difficulties associated with the transition out of communism—and continues today after a one-year interruption in 1990. Between 1989 and 1996 life expectancy in the Czech Republic increased 2.3 years for males and 1.8 years for females, thereby demonstrating that the Czechs are escaping the general Eastern European trend in mortality (Institute of Health Information and Statistics of the Czech Republic 1997; Rychtaříková 1996).

It can therefore be argued that the Czech Republic has experienced stressful events like its neighbors, but has seen male mortality generally fall instead of rise in the last decade. Declines in deaths from heart disease, stroke, and cirrhosis of the liver for 25- to 44-year-old males and in heart and respiratory diseases for 45- to 59-year-old males are principal causes of the Czech downturn in mortality. Consequently, American and Czech demographers Elwood Carlson and Jitka Rychtaříková (1996:9) reject a stress hypothesis for the Czech Republic by pointing out that "rapid declines in nearly all causes of death for all age groups after 1990 has coincided with rapid social transformation, economic insecurity, stress, unemployment, new freedom in the marketplace to buy and sell an unprecedented variety of foodstuffs, and in general, an acceleration of the sort of 'westernization' that was supposed to be producing rising death rates."

Thus, the question remains unanswered: Were significant numbers of people in the former Soviet Union and Eastern Europe, primarily middle-aged men, so stressed by their circumstances that increasingly higher proportions of them succumbed to heart attacks over a period of 30 years? Although there is a possibility that East-West differences in cardiovascular mortality are linked to chronically stressful socioeconomic and psychological conditions, German sociologist Johannes Siegrist (1996:169) finds that "while suggestive, no direct empirical evidence so far exists to confirm such a link." The social stress explanation of increased mortality needs evidence to support its role as the primary social determinant. To claim that communism stressed middle-aged working-class men so severely that they dropped dead from heart ailments does not seem highly likely. It may be that the stress has a more indirect effect and influences life expectancy by promoting unhealthy lifestyles.

HEALTH LIFESTYLES

The health lifestyles explanation lays the blame for poor health upon unhealthy practices and social conditions. Health lifestyles are collective patterns of health-related behavior based on choices from options available to people according to their life chances (Cockerham and Ritchey 1997; Cockerham, Rütten, and Abel 1997). These life chances include the effects of age, gender, race/ethnicity, and other variables that affect lifestyle choices. The behaviors that are generated from these choices can have either positive or negative consequences on body and mind, but nonetheless form an overall pattern of health practices that constitute a lifestyle.

Life Choices versus Life Chances

Sociological thinking on lifestyles generally remains guided by the insight of the renowned German sociologist Max Weber ([1922] 1978). Weber's work, as expressed in his 1922 classic, *Economy and Society*, suggests that lifestyles have two major components: (1) life choice (self-direction) and (2) life chances (the structural probabilities of acquiring satisfaction). His most important contribution toward conceptualizing lifestyles is identification of the dialectical interplay between choice and chance in lifestyle determination (Cockerham, Abel, and Lüschen 1993). Individuals have a range of freedom, but not complete freedom in choosing a lifestyle. That is, people are not entirely free to determine their lifestyle but have the freedom to choose within the social constraints that apply to their situation in life.

While this perspective suggests that participation in a healthy lifestyle—which typically involves decisions about food, exercise, coping with stress, smoking, alcohol and drug use, risk of infection and accidents, and physical appearance—is largely up to the individual, the author and his colleagues (Cockerham et al. 1997) indicate that this may not necessarily be the case. Structural constraints embedded in life chances may be the dominant factor in the operationalization of health lifestyles. Although Weber's perspective favors choice over chance, he recognizes the central role of chance in lifestyle selection. Life chances, in a Weberian context, are anchored in structural conditions that are largely socioeconomic—like income, property, and the opportunity for profit—but also involve rights, norms, and probabilities that other people will respond to in a certain way (Dahrendorf 1979). Thus, Weber does not consider life chances to be pure chance; rather, they are the chances people have in life because of their social circumstances to satisfy their needs and desires. People with the desires and the means may choose; those lacking in some way cannot choose so easily and may find their lifestyle determined more by external circumstances.

However, the author and his associates (Cockerham et al. 1997) find that chance is even more of a determining factor in lifestyle selection than Weber allows. Drawing upon the work of Pierre Bourdieu (1977, 1984) and his concept of habitus, they assign priority to chance over choice—although choice remains important. Bourdieu (1984), for example, notes that categories of perception—the basis for self-direction—are largely determined by socialization, experience, and the reality of class circumstances. The habitus, a mind-set that guides social action, is limited by its perceptual boundaries. The dispositions produced are typically compatible with the constraints imposed by the larger social order, and set the individual on a stable and consistent course of action. These constraints may in fact leave people with little or no choice in exposing themselves to unhealthy conditions and practices.

In societies, like those in the former socialist countries, where people lack information about health and have little control over their diet, ecological pollution, or a social environment where smoking and heavy drinking is normative, poor health lifestyles are likely. Andrew Nagorski (1993) reports that Eastern Europeans are among the world's heaviest drinkers and smokers, and their diet is loaded with fat. Vodka and cigarettes were cheap under Communism and easily available in large quantities, and the average citizen had little choice about which foods to purchase and consume. Nagorski (1993:189) states: "If Eastern Europeans seemed less concerned about maintaining health habits, if they shrugged off warnings about the dangers of drinking, smoking, and lack of exercise more easily than their Western counterparts, if they seemed to take ecological devastation more fatalistically, this was a natural result of the sense of powerlessness the communist system encouraged at every turn."

British social scientist Peggy Watson (1995) has argued, however, that lifestyle factors are not the primary cause of the rising mortality in Eastern Europe. She claims that Eastern Europeans do not eat more animal fat, smoke more cigarettes, or drink more alcohol than people in Western Europe. "They may well," states Watson (1995:927), "eat, smoke and drink more than is good for their health—the point is that they do not seem to be unique in this respect." Yet current East-West comparisons do not support Watson's conclusions. In a major study in Eastern Europe, Czech researcher Antonin Kubik and an international team of associates (Kubik et al. 1995) found that cigarette sales increased significantly throughout the region in the 1960s and 1970s. "By the 1980s," state Kubik and his colleagues (1995:2456), "the dramatic increases in lung cancer mortality rates in the [Eastern European] countries resulted in rates that often well exceed [those in the West]." Over 90% of these deaths were caused by smoking. In Russia, the number of cigarettes imported into the country doubled between 1965 and 1989 to more than 73 billion per year, making the nation the largest importer of cigarettes in the world (Hurt 1995). The prevalence of smoking varies by region in Russia, with smoking rates for males in industrial areas as high as 78.6% in 1986. For the adult population as a whole, the prevalence of smoking rose from 53% in 1985 to 67% in 1992 (Hurt 1995; Tchachenko and Riazantsev 1993). While smoking was decreasing in the West, it was increasing in the East (Kubik et al. 1995).

As for alcohol use, there is ample evidence that drinking has continued to increase in Russia to the point, as will be discussed, that the Russians now consume more hard liquor than any other country in the world. Alcohol consumption in Poland and other Eastern European countries has likewise become a health hazard beyond that of any Western country (Okólski 1993). Data on fat consumption are inconclusive. Watson claims that fat intake has increased in Eastern Europe, but finds consumption levels somewhat below the West. However, as she observes, her data source does not differentiate between types of fat consumed. Saturated fats, which increase cholesterol levels, are the most dangerous to health, and are found in animal fats, foods of animal origin (e.g., egg yolks), and hydrogenated shortenings like palm and coconut oil. In contrast, unsaturated fats like corn, cottonseed, and sunflower oil tend to *lower* serum cholesterol; monounsaturated fats, like olive and peanut oil, neither raise nor lower cholesterol. Findings based only on overall levels of fat consumption without differentiating between types of fat cannot convey accurate assessments.

Watson (1995:927) also relies on a German survey (Lüschen and Apelt 1992) which she claims "has provided further and more detailed evidence of slightly 'healthier' eating habits among East Germans than among West Germans." Yet this survey had only two questionnaire items on food habits (Likert-type statements of agreement-disagreement), and thus cannot be considered an in-depth analysis. Moreover, Nagorski (1993) has reported on the poor quality of the care of livestock and the condition of food in Eastern Europe, while in Russia there is evidence that the quality and quantity of nutrition declined between 1989 and 1992 (Rush and Welch 1996). Overall, it appears that diets in the former socialist countries were less healthy than the Western equivalent, not only in regard to fatty meat but also for a lack of fresh vegetables and fruit in the winter (Hungarian Central Statistical Office 1995; Keep 1995; Rush and Welch 1996; Tulchinsky and Varavikova 1996).

While Watson's research on rising mortality among Eastern European men provides valuable insight in a number of areas, her argument regarding lifestyles is unconvincing. She seems to regard lifestyles largely as a matter of choice, and since such choices were constrained by communism, they were not the major determinant of the downturn in life expectancy. Citing the work of British sociologist Anthony Giddens (1991), Watson suggests that individual lifestyle choices are largely a product of modernity and emerge in greater force when tradition loses its hold on society. She argues, however, that tradition was becoming more entrenched in Eastern Europe under communism, coping strategies were fixed, and lifestyle choices intended to create a new stage of life were unavailable. That is, lifestyle choices were limited to making the best of the life that was available, rather than implementing the lifestyle one desired. "Choices made at the level of the individual," comments Watson (1995:933), "were socially structured by the resources and options available, and the perceptual frameworks to which such arrangements gave rise." Yet this is exactly the point. Lifestyles in the former socialist countries were shaped primarily by life chances (structure) and not life choices. To focus more or less exclusively on choice overlooks the potentially dominant role of chance in lifestyle selection. The link between choice and lifestyles has been overemphasized in most interpretations of Weber, while the connection between lifestyles and life chances has received scant attention (Cockerham et al. 1993).

The major argument against the lifestyle explanation is that it places responsibility for health directly on the individual and his or her lifestyle choices; i.e., when people develop poor health or die prematurely it is their fault because of these choices. This allows the capitalist system and its health care sector to escape blame for unhealthy social conditions or medical mistakes (Navarro 1986; Waitzkin 1983). Consequently, the lifestyle explanation is depicted as a form of "blaming the victim," which permits the state and powerful groups to evade responsibility. There is some justification for this view if lifestyles are considered to be more or less exclusively based on individual choice; however, there is little empirical evidence that lifestyles are merely a deliberate product of independent individuals. As Bourdieu (Bourdieu and Wacquant 1992:183) explains: "Autonomy does not come without the social conditions of autonomy and these conditions cannot be obtained on an individual basis." Therefore, as noted, life chances and the parameters they set for choice selection play an especially powerful role in determining lifestyles (Cockerham et al. 1997).

If life chances constrain life choices in the more consumption-oriented and individualistic West, they are likely to impose even greater limits on lifestyle choices in the East. During the Soviet era, for example, high-quality foodstuffs were not widely available in Russia (Chamberlain 1982). The food consumed was determined more by what was available than by personal choice over a range of options. Although the diet was nutritionally adequate, it was unbalanced by an excess of carbohydrates and fatty meats, shortages in fresh fruits and vegetables in winter months, and a lack of variety (Keep 1995; Knaus 1981; Rush and Welch 1996; Tulchinsky and Varavikova 1996). We would argue that such external constraints (life chances) dominate choices and result in relatively unhealthy lifestyle patterns and rising mortality.

Support for the Lifestyle Explanation

Evidence supporting a lifestyle explanation for the rise in mortality comes from at least four sources: (1) prior research, (2) the types of disease most responsible for the increase, (3) Russia's anti-alcohol campaign, and (4) recent surveys of health behavior. First, several studies and research reports suggest that unhealthy lifestyles are the major cause of the rise in mortality in the former Soviet Union and Eastern Europe in general (Adevi et al. 1997; Cockerham 1997; Eberstadt 1990; Feachem 1994; Kulin and Skakkeback 1995; Wnuk-Lipinski and Illsley 1990) and in the former Czechoslovakia (Janečková and Hnilicová 1992) and Poland (World Bank 1992) in particular. Second, a particularly strong association exists between cardiovascular diseases and health lifestyle practices involving diet, exercise, smoking, and heavy drinking (Cockerham 1998), and, as previously discussed, the leading overall causes of the mortality increase in Russia and Eastern Europe are diseases of the circulatory system. The increase in heart disease would suggest an increase in risk behavior; and this appears to be the case based on data showing a dramatic rise in the per capita consumption of cigarettes and hard liquor in Eastern Europe between the mid-1960s and mid-1980s (Eberstadt 1990), increasingly higher levels of alcohol consumption in Russia between 1971–84 and 1987–93 (Shkolnikov and Nemtsov 1994), and a rise in the percentage of regular smokers in Hungary between 1984 and 1994 (Antal 1994; Hungarian Central Statistical Office 1996). Moreover, in Hungary, deaths from cirrhosis of the liver and the estimated number of alcoholics doubled between 1987 and 1993 (Hungarian Ministry of Welfare 1995). Third, while not conclusive, the relationship between a lifestyle involving heavy alcohol use and the rise in male mortality appears especially important. As Okólski (1993:177) puts it: "It seems that of all plausible determinants of adult male mortality increase in Eastern Europe, the most widely accepted underlying factor is growing alcohol consumption." A strong relationship between alcohol consumption and decreased male life expectancy has been found in both Eastern Europe (Okólski 1993) and Russia (Anderson and Silver 1990; Meslé and Shkolnikov 1995; Meslé, Shkolnikov, and Vallin 1992; Ponarin 1996; Shkolnikov and Nemtsov 1994).

The magnitude of alcohol use in the former Soviet Union is illustrated by the fact that tax revenues from sales of vodka accounted for 35% of the Soviet budget in 1988. By 1995, vodka generated less than 5% of revenues, not because of decreased consumption, but because of the government's loss of the state monopoly on production and sales and its inability to control the black market. In 1995, Russians consumed 4.1 gallons of hard liquor per capita—the highest in the world. In an extensive study of the alcohol-mortality relationship in Russia, Vladimir Shkolnikov and Alexander Nemtsov (1994) investigated alcohol sales and consumption between 1971 and 1993. Their focus was on Gorbachev's 1984–87 anti-alcohol campaign, and they determined that both reported and real alcohol consumption declined during this period. Calculating the difference between observed and expected deaths by sex and age, Shkolnikov and Nemtsov found that longevity increased 3.2 years for males and 1.3 years for females during the campaign's duration, with the greatest advances occurring in 1986. Shkolnikov and Nemtsov (1994:1) conclude that "the rapid mortality decrease in the years 1984 to 1987 can be assumed to reflect a pure effect of reduced alcohol abuse on mortality, because there were no other significant changes in conditions of the public health in that short period." The fact that alcohol abuse was very much a regional (or ethnic) problem (Keep 1995:269) may help explain why the rise in adult male mortality has been greater in Russia and the Baltic states (where consumption was highest) than in Central Asia.

According to Shkolnikov and Nemtsov (1994), the mode of drinking common to middle-aged Slavic males is part of a northern European lifestyle involving rapid group consumption of large doses of vodka with a light snack—the participant is expected to continue to drink with his fellows even when he feels he has had enough. Apparently little or no social stigma is associated with drunkenness. Earlier in the twentieth century Russian workers typically drank large amounts of alcohol only on their days off (Sundays and Russian Orthodox Church holidays). However, during the Soviet period, heavy alcohol consumption became common throughout the year, which most likely fostered a lifestyle characterized by consistent binge drinking. This situation suggests that it is the normative demands of a particular lifestyle, rather than health policy or stress, that is primarily responsible for the pattern of male drinking in Russia.

For example, in a comparison of health-related behavior in Helsinki and Moscow, Finnish sociologist Hannele Palosuo and her Finnish and Russian colleagues (Palosuo et al. 1995) found that over 89% of both the Finns and the Russians reported they drank alcohol. The Finns, in fact, share a similar drinking style and exceedingly high level of per capita consumption of alcohol with the Russians. However, Palosuo and her associates found that dramatically higher percentages of men (35%) and women (41%) in their Moscow sample did not exercise as a health-promoting activity. In Helsinki, in stark contrast, practically all respondents reported some physical exercise intended to benefit their health. Finns were also significantly more likely to eat a healthy diet, get sufficient sleep and rest, and avoid harmful drugs. The Finns likewise rated their diet as being more healthy than the Russian respondents. Russians were more likely to have regular medical checkups from a physician, but this likely resulted from mandatory requirements to have such exams. In Moscow some 46% of the men and only 16% of the women respondents were smokers compared to 35% of the men and 25% of the women in Helsinki. Consequently, the highest concentration of smokers was found among Moscow males. Except for drinking, which is a serious problem in both countries, the Finns show a much healthier lifestyle than the Russians—especially Russian men. They also live longer, with 1996 statistics showing that Finnish male life expectancy was 73.8 years (compared to 59.6 years for Russian males) and Finnish female longevity was 77.2 years (compared to 72.7 years for Russian females).

Other evidence supporting a lifestyle explanation for rising mortality is found in Hungary's 1994 health behavior survey (Hungarian Central Statistical Office 1995). This nationwide survey of 5,476 households (an 85% response rate) found that the percentage of smokers had increased to 35% from 31.9% in 1986. Some 72% of the sample drank alcohol regularly, with 11.6% characterized as "excessive drinkers." Only 21.4% of the men and 13.5% of the women reported regular physical exercise, while less than 10% of the men and 12.5% of the women ate vegetables almost every day in the winter. Furthermore, over half of all visits to physicians were made by just 10% of the respondents. Hungary's health profile is among the worst in Eastern Europe, and these data help us to understand why. For example, Hungary's mortality rate rose from 10.2 deaths per 1,000 persons in 1960 to 14.3 in 1994 with the rise in heart disease among middle-aged men serving as the principal cause (Carlson 1989; Hungarian Central Statistical Office 1996; Józan 1989, 1996b; Nagorski 1993).

Although Soviet-style health policy and social stress have likely contributed to the downturn in life expectancy in Russia and Eastern Europe, this review of the evidence suggests that unhealthy lifestyles are the primary social determinant of the higher death rates and currently offer the most promising line of inquiry for future research.

Chapter 3

Health Lifestyles:
A Theoretical Perspective

Since lifestyles are the most likely primary social determinant of the downturn in longevity in the former socialist countries, it is necessary to discover why this is the case. The initial step in this process is to present a theoretical perspective to guide subsequent discussion. As defined in the last chapter, health lifestyles are collective patterns of health-related behavior based on choices from options available to people according to their life chances. Consequently, the behaviors that people select which affect their health, either positively or negatively, are not simply random acts of individuals but constitute a recognizable pattern of activities specific to certain groups, social strata, and societies.

Investigating this situation not only helps explain the rise in mortality in the former Soviet bloc, but also addresses a fundamental debate in sociology and other social sciences over the relative contributions of structure and agency. Structure refers to the collective patterns associated with societies, institutions, social classes, communities, groups, and roles that both constrain and enable individuals, while agency is the freely chosen activities of individuals. Structures, then, can be conceptualized as sets of mutually sustaining schemas (rules) and resources that empower and constrain social action and tend to be reproduced by that action (Sewell 1992:19). Agency, in contrast, is a process in which individuals—influenced by their past but also oriented toward the future (as a capacity to image alternative possibilities) and the present (as a capacity to consider both past habits and future situations within the contingencies of the moment)—critically evaluate and choose their course of action (Emirbayer and Mische 1998:963). Clearly, structure and agency are interactive. Structure either enables or constrains individuals from social practices that they have chosen (or wish to choose) through a process of agency, while agency, in turn, reproduces structure when the practices it has activated are continued. No contemporary theoretical perspective denies that either structure or agency is important; rather, the debate centers on the extent to which one or the other may be dominant. Proponents of structure emphasize the power of structural conditions in determining social behavior, while advocates of agency note the ability of actors to choose their behavior and act on their own regardless of structural constraints.

I will begin the discussion with an examination of the concept of lifestyles which includes a review of the early-twentieth-century work of Max Weber. Weber is particularly important because he focuses on the broad displacement of European society at the turn of the last century. In fact, Weber has been described as standing between a vanishing and rising era (Jaspers 1988). In his time, industrial society was rising, while traditional society—based on the last vestiges of European feudalism— was vanishing. Weber's own early studies of the urban migration of German agricultural workers from the Prussian estates east of the river Elbe and the decline of the centuries-old domination by the region's landed aristocracy—the Junkers—demonstrated a process of irreversible social change (Mommsen 1989). However, just as modernization dissolved the structure of feudal society and created the industrial age, modernization today has changed industrial society, and another modernity is coming into being (Beck 1992). A major casualty of this change is socialism, whose European communist variant was too rigid, repressive, and stagnant in coping with this emerging new modernity.

Regardless of whether we call this oncoming period high modernity (Giddens 1991), reflexive modernity (Beck 1992), or postmodernity (Bauman 1992; Bertens 1995; Smart 1992, 1993), we are witnessing a new modernity that is moving well beyond its classical industrial model. I will therefore turn to the work of two contemporary sociological theorists—Anthony Giddens and Pierre Bourdieu—to provide insight into recent social conditions. Next I apply their work to health lifestyles and discuss the implications for the former socialist countries.

THE LIFESTYLES CONCEPT

One of the most important new developments in sociological theory is the increased attention given to lifestyles as a key concept in explaining human social behavior (Abel 1991; Chaney 1996; Giddens 1991; Maffesoli 1996). Lifestyles are utilitarian social practices and ways of living adopted by individuals which reflect personal, group, and socioeconomic identities (Giddens 1991). Stated simply, lifestyles help us make sense of what people do, why they do it, and what doing it means to them and others (Chaney 1996). Basically, lifestyles are forms of consumerism involving preferences in food, bodily dress and appearance, housing, work habits, leisure, and other status-oriented behavior that differentiates between people. Health lifestyles, for example, are a subtype of lifestyles generally. They can be healthy or unhealthy and consist of actions involving eating habits, drinking, smoking, exercise, coping with stress, relaxation, personal hygiene, and other health-related behavior. While such lifestyles are oriented toward producing health, the aim of the activity is ultimately toward its consumption as people try to be healthy so they can *use* their health to live longer, enjoy life, feel and/or look good, be able to keep on working, and the like (Cockerham 1998).

While it might be presumed that lifestyles, health or otherwise, are common only to the affluent or would-be affluent, this is not the case. All individuals, groups, and social classes have a particular lifestyle that reflects their pattern of consumption (Chaney 1996; Giddens 1991). Differences are matters of resources, taste, and style, but even the socially and economically disadvantaged have distinct lifestyles. As Giddens (1991:86) points out: "Lifestyle habits are constructed through the resistances of ghetto life as well as through the direct elaboration of distinctive cultural styles and modes of activity." Furthermore, lifestyles sometimes cross social boundaries and become broadly representative of a large number of people in a society (Chaney 1996). The best example in Weber's (1958) work is his analysis of the manner in which the Protestant ethic became part of Western culture and influenced the rise of capitalism as a generally shared belief system. Consequently, certain lifestyles not only set people apart, but also can be incorporated into the mainstream culture of society.

Given the massive social, economic, technological, and political changes that have taken place in the late twentieth century, lifestyles have gained particular significance as individual and collective expressions of differences and similarities. Some sociologists have even argued that lifestyle situations and milieus are becoming more important influences on group behavior than social class (Hradil 1987). The extent to which this is the case remains uncertain, but it is nonetheless clear that there is a growing interest in lifestyle research (Abel 1991; Chaney 1996; Giddens 1991). As Italian sociologist Michel Maffesoli (1996) explains, the term "lifestyles" can no longer be given cursory treatment because of the resurgence of interest in the concept.

Max Weber

Among the classical theorists, Weber provides the deepest insight into the lifestyle concept. Weber ([1922]1978:932) linked lifestyles to status by pointing out that a distinguishing characteristic of status is "status honor or prestige which is normally expressed by the fact that above all else a specific *style of life* is expected from all those who wish to belong to the circle." Status, not class, plays the larger role in Weber's perspective. Weber views class strictly as a reflection of the marketplace, signifying a person's level of income, property, or economic skill. Status groups, on the other hand, are aggregates of people with similar status, class backgrounds, and political influence, and they originate through a sharing of similar lifestyles or as a means to preserve a particular style of life. Weber made the pertinent observation that lifestyles are based not so much on what a person produces, but on what he or she consumes. As Weber ([1922]1978:933) puts it: "one might thus say that classes are stratified according to their relations to the production and acquisition of goods: whereas status groups are stratified according to the principles of their *consumption* of goods as represented by special styles of life."

Consumption is, of course, not independent of production; rather, lifestyle differences between status groups are based on their relationship to the means of consumption, not the means of production. The economic mode of production sets the basic parameters within which consumption occurs, but does not determine or even necessarily affect specific forms of it (Bocock 1993). This is because the consumption of goods and services conveys a social meaning that displays, at the time, the status and social identity of the consumer. Consumption can therefore be regarded as a set of social and cultural practices that *establish* differences between groups, not merely a means of *expressing* differences that are already in place because of economic factors (Bocock 1993:64; Bourdieu 1984). It is the use of particular goods and services through distinct lifestyles that ultimately distinguishes status groups from one another.

Three terms in the original German are used by Weber to express his concept of lifestyles. These terms are *Stilisierung des Lebens* (stylization of life) or, more simply, *Lebensstil* (lifestyle), along with *Lebensführung* (life conduct) and *Lebenschancen* (life chances), which comprise the two basic components of lifestyles (Abel and Cockerham 1993; Cockerham, Abel, and Lüschen 1993). *Lebensführung* refers to the choices that people have in their selection of lifestyles and *Lebenschancen* is the probability of realizing those choices. This major distinction in Weber's concept of lifestyles has been obscured in English-language translations of his *Wirtschaft und Gesellschaft* ([1922]1978). In Gerth and Mills (Weber 1946) and Roth and Wittch (Weber [1922]1978)—the most frequently cited English versions—*Stilisierung des Lebens* and *Lebensführung* are both mutually translated as "lifestyles." Yet, *Lebensführung*, translated literally, means life conduct and refers to choice or self-direction in behavior, not lifestyles.

British sociologist Ralf Dahrendorf (1979:73) notes that while Weber is vague about what he means by life chances, the best interpretation is that life chances are "the crystallized probability of finding satisfaction for interests, wants, and needs, thus the probability of the occurrence of events which bring about satisfaction." The probability of acquiring satisfaction is anchored in structural conditions that are largely economic, but Dahrendorf suggests the concept of life chances also involves rights, norms, and social relationships (the probability that others will respond in a certain manner). Weber does not consider life chances to be a matter of pure chance; rather, they are the chances people have in life because of their social situation. His overall thesis is that chance is socially determined and social structure is an arrangement of chances. Hence, lifestyles are not random behaviors unrelated to structure, but typically are deliberate choices influenced by life chances.

Consequently, the author and his colleagues (Cockerham et al. 1993) point out that Weber's most important contribution to conceptualizing lifestyles in sociological terms is to impose a dialectical capstone over the interplay of choice and chance in lifestyle determination. Choices and the constraints of life chances work off of one another to determine a distinctive lifestyle for individuals and groups. This view is consistent with the Hegelian concept of thesis, antithesis, and synthesis which influenced Weber's intellectual development, although his focus was more on the nature of dialectic exchanges than a search for a grand synthesis in the German tradition (Münch 1988, 1993).

The identification of life chances as the dialectic opposite of choice in Weber's lifestyle scheme provides the theoretical key to conceptualizing the manner in which lifestyles are operationalized in the empirical world. It can be said that individuals have a range of freedom, yet not complete freedom, in choosing a lifestyle. That is, people are not entirely free in determining their lifestyle but have the freedom to choose within the social constraints that apply to their situation in life. Lifestyle constraints, in a Weberian context, are primarily socioeconomic in origin. Therefore, the value of Weber's concept is that it can account for the interplay of individual choice and structural constraints in operationalizing a lifestyle.

However, despite his emphasis on choice, Weber did not view patterns of social action as the uncoordinated practices of individuals. Rather, he saw them as regularities and uniformities repeated by numerous actors over time. The ways in which individuals act in concert, not as single actors, are the focus of his attention (Kalberg 1994). For example, Weber suggests that the "spirit" of capitalism was not uniquely Western, nor particularly unusual if considered merely an attribute of individuals. He suggests that there have always been economically successful people who conducted their business on a systematic basis, had frugal personal habits, worked harder than their employees, and invested their earnings (Bendix 1960:54–5). But, as individuals, they could not establish a dominant economic system like capitalism. "In order that a manner of life so well adapted to the peculiarities of capitalism could be selected at all," states Weber (1958:55), "i.e. should come to dominate others, it had to originate somewhere, and not in isolated individuals alone, but as a way of life common to whole groups of men [and women]."

It is the origin of this lifestyle which Weber insists requires attention, and he finds it in the Protestant ethic of the early Calvinists, whom he credits for the expansion of modern capitalism. Weber (1958:174) argues that the influence of the Puritan outlook is "much more important than the mere encouragement of capital accumulation—it favored the development of a rational bourgeois economic life" which stands "at the cradle" of the modern economic person. Thus, the transformation of individual action into collective patterns of behavior is Weber's focal point of analysis. The bridge from agency to structure for Weber is the "ideal type" which allowed him to make general statements about structural processes or entities, such as the Protestant ethic, bureaucracy, authority, rationality, and the major world religions (Kalberg 1994; Mommsen 1989; Smelser 1988).

Although Weber recognizes the constraining effects of structure, such as his warning of the potential for bureaucratic organizations to suppress freedom of action by the individual, he ultimately favors the capacity of the individual to assume control over his or her circumstances (Alexander 1987; Löwith 1982; Mommsen 1989; Roth 1987). Whereas the individual may not be capable of breaking the iron cage of bureaucratic submission for all, he or she can break it for themselves by finding ways to maneuver around its barriers (Löwith 1982). Weber (1949:124–5) observes, for instance, that people associate the strongest feelings of freedom with those actions in which they pursue a clear purpose and accomplish rationally with the most adequate means at their disposal. All social action, in Weber's view, takes place in contexts that imply both constraints and opportunities, with the actor's interpretive understanding (*Verstehen*) of the situation guiding interaction (Kalberg 1994).

Therefore, when Weber discusses lifestyles, his basic approach is to understand the subjective meanings individuals attach to their choices and the ways in which these meanings are transformed into collective patterns of behavior. Weber's lifestyle concept can account for individual choice and structural constraints, thus merging the functions of both structure and agency. Although the notion of "lifestyle" was a marginal idea in his discussion of status groups, Weber provides a basic framework for conceptualizing its basic parameters. His overall contribution to our understanding of contemporary lifestyles is that lifestyles (1) are associated with status groups, and therefore are principally a collective rather than an individual phenomenon; (2) represent patterns of consumption, not production; and (3) are shaped by the dialectical interplay between life choices and life chances, with choice playing the greater role.

Anthony Giddens

Giddens (1991) describes how modernity—the mode of social life resulting from the Industrial Revolution—influences contemporary lifestyles. He explains that modernity differs from all previous forms of social order because of its dynamism, global impact, and the degree to which it undercuts traditional customs and habits. The more tradition loses its hold, observes Giddens, the more individuals are forced to negotiate lifestyle choices among a variety of local and, increasingly, global options.

Consequently, modernity promotes a diversity of lifestyle choices, and even people in the lowest social classes have some choice because, in Giddens's view, no culture eliminates choice altogether in day-to-day affairs.

However, Giddens does not overlook the influence of sources external to the individual on lifestyle choices, and cites group pressures, role models, and socioeconomic conditions as examples. In conditions of high modernity, people are likely to be pushed by social situations into choosing a particular lifestyle, or as Giddens (1991:81) puts it, "we have no choice but to choose." That is, it is necessary to adopt the appropriate lifestyle of a specific group or stratum of society if one wishes to belong to it and move within it. Giddens (1991:82) makes the pertinent observation that "a lifestyle involves a cluster of habits and orientations, and hence has a certain unity—important to a continuing sense of ontological security—that connects options to a more or less ordered pattern." As a result, the particular lifestyle choices an individual makes tend to fit a pattern which makes alternative choices be "out of character." The basic message is that lifestyles not only fulfill utilitarian needs but provide material form to one's self-identity.

Giddens takes the position that lifestyles occur within the constraints and opportunities provided by an individual's social location, but everyone—to some extent—is forced to adopt reflexivity-constructed lifestyles to sustain his or her self-identity (Shillling 1993). This reflexivity is grounded in a climate of change resulting from society's evolution into high modernity. Giddens's (1991) work provides an introduction to new conditions, noting how transformations of time and space, combined with certain disembedding systems like increasingly sophisticated and abstract money systems and the penetration of technical knowledge throughout society, promote constant change. Giddens finds that as social life becomes more open, the contexts for action more plural, and authority more diverse, lifestyle choices are increasingly more important in the construction of self-identity and daily activities.

Another area of Giddens's (1984) work relevant to lifestyle theory is his notion of the duality of structure as the centerpiece of his structuration theory. Giddens explains that neither structure nor agency are independent of each other; rather, they are codependent. Structure is not possible without action because action reproduces structure. Action is not possible without structure because action begins with a given structure resulting from prior actions. An agent is not the abstract or dependent subject of action but an individual who constructs social behavior. That behavior, however, is embedded in a structure and contributes to that structure's continuation or change. Structures are therefore not pre-determined but evolve through social interaction. Since structures are both the means and outcomes of action, they contain a duality dimension; that is, structures are both objective (constraining) and subjective (enabling) at the same time.

The logical appeal of Giddens's notion of the duality of structure is based on his recognition that structures empower agents as well as constrain them and, in the process, can be changed by the practices of those agents. This insight helps to overcome arguments that structures are rigid, impervious to agency, and impossible to change, while assigning agents the capacity for innovation and improvisation. Giddens does note that structures place limits on the range of options open to an actor or plurality of actors in particular circumstances. Moreover, he acknowledges that it is possible for the structured properties of social systems to stretch out in time and space to the point at which they are beyond the control of any individual actors. Nevertheless, he strongly favors agency over structure. Giddens (1984:129), in fact, claims that there is no such entity as a distinctive type of "structural explanation" in the social sciences, and maintains that "all explanations will involve at least implicit reference both to the purposive, reasoning behavior of agents and to its intersection with constraining and enabling features of the social and material contexts of that behavior."

In Giddens's (1991) view, lifestyles are structured patterns of behavior with norms, values, and boundaries, yet through the feedback processes of social agents they are reproduced or transformed over time as people operationalize them. Whereas structure may hinder the creativity of agents in constructing or modifying lifestyles, agents have the capacity to change structures and are ultimately viewed as the stronger entity. What we primarily gain from Giddens's analysis is the recognition of (1) late or high modernity's role in fostering a diversity of lifestyle choices; (2) the necessity of having to choose; (3) the tendency of choices to cluster into distinct patterns; (4) the role played by lifestyles in expressing self-identity for the individual; and (5) the dual nature of structure.

Pierre Bourdieu

Whereas Weber and Giddens favor agency in the agency-structure debate, Bourdieu favors structure. Bourdieu's principal focus is on the question of how routine practices of individuals are influenced by the external structure of their social world and how these practices, conversely, contribute to the maintenance of that structure (Jenkins 1992). The key concept in this regard is that of "habitus," which Bourdieu (1990:53) defines as "systems of durable, transposable dispositions, structured structures predisposed to operate as structuring structures, that is, as principles which generate and organize practices and representations that can be objectively adapted to their outcomes without presupposing a conscious aiming at ends or an express mastery of the operations necessary in order to attain them." Thus, Bourdieu maintains that knowledge of social structures and conditions produce enduring orientations toward action that are more or less routine, and when these orientations are acted upon they tend to reproduce the structures from which they are derived.

The lasting nature of the orientations and control imposed by habitus on thought, perception, and action signals a dominant role for structure in guiding social behavior. As Bourdieu (Bourdieu and Wacquant 1992) explains, the human mind is socially bounded and constructed within the limits of experience, upbringing, and training. People are able to assess their circumstances, but their perceptions are typically shaped by their particular social and economic conditions. "The *habitus*," states Bourdieu (1990:54), ". . . ensures the active presence of past experiences, which, deposited in each organism in the form of schemes of perception, thought and action, tend to guarantee the 'correctness' of practices and their constancy over time, more reliably than all formal rules and explicit norms." Therefore, habitus provides a cognitive map of an individual's social world and channels behavior down paths that appear to be reasonable to the individual and society.

However, situations vary—so habitus can vary to fit the situation. Habitus is not, in Bourdieu's view, a mechanical response to all situations; rather, the dispositions it reflects are subject to change by the individual. The same habitus can generate different, even opposite outcomes, since people are not mechanically pushed about by external forces but are able to act on their own. Bourdieu (1977), in fact, calls for the abandonment of theories that explicitly or implicitly treat social practices as mechanical reactions to situations or roles. But he maintains that rejection of mechanistic theories does not imply that we should bestow on some creative free will the power to determine the meaning of situations and the intentions of actors. The dispositions generated by habitus tend to be compatible with constraints set by society through experience, socialization, and the realities of class circumstances; therefore, usual modes of behaving—not unpredictable novelty—typically prevail.

Bourdieu's conceptualization of habitus as a mind-set that operates more or less routinely, even unconsciously, to guide behavior has prompted critics like American sociologist Jeffrey Alexander (1995) to argue that habitus has no independent power to direct action. Alexander (1995:136), calling habitus a "Trojan horse for determinism," claims it is a reflection and replication of exterior structures rather than a locus for voluntary action. The habitus, in Alexander's view, merely translates exterior social structures into subjective constraints in a noninterpretive way. This places actors in a continuous adaptation to their external environment instead of in a state of discourse with it. What the habitus initiates, states Alexander (1995:138), "is an endless and circular account of objective structures structuring subjective structures that structure objective structures in turn." Because it does not have its own emergent properties, internal complexity, and logic, Alexander concludes that the habitus has no real independence and cannot be a means of establishing a true micro-macro link between the individual and society in accounting for social behavior.

Yet, is this really the case? Certainly Bourdieu's concept of habitus can suggest an endless and circular routine of structure structuring structures that lacks the properties, complexity, and logical pathways seen in Sigmund Freud's notion of the personality or George Herbert Mead's concept of self. But the habitus does provide a relatively seamless blending of macro and micro processes by assimilating exterior structures into the subjectivity of the individual and providing a general frame of reference, with boundaries and constraints, for the conduct of everyday life. The habitus generates perceptual schemes that promote consistent and routine forms of behavior; it also, as Bourdieu regularly insists, reorients the agent toward new or modified behaviors when social situations require change. The habitus accounts best for routine and day-to-day behaviors grounded in normative structures that require little thinking and adjustment, but it nevertheless has the capacity for creative direction. Habitus is also a strategy-generating entity that enables agents to cope with unforeseen and changing circumstances and, in Bourdieu's (1977) view, makes possible the achievement of an infinite diversity of tasks. As Bourdieu (Bourdieu and Wacquant 1992:133) explains: "habitus is not the fate that some people read into it"; as a product of history, "it is an *open system of dispositions* that is constantly subjected to experiences and therefore constantly affected by them in a way that either reinforces or modifies its structures."

Bourdieu (Bourdieu and Wacquant 1992:135) therefore rejects the notion that his scheme is overly deterministic, but he assigns a strong preference to structure in influencing behavior. In his view, people can consciously inhibit or alter their dispositions, but categories of perception and appreciation—the basis for self-determination—are themselves largely determined by socialization and experience, which includes recognition of the reality of their class situation. In Bourdieu's concept, social practices are based upon *both* the objective structures that define external constraints affecting interaction, and the immediate lived experience of agents which shape internal categories of perception and appreciation; however, while the two components are equally necessary, they are not equal (Wacquant 1992:11). When it comes to the extent to which dispositions to act are socially determined, Bourdieu (Bourdieu and Wacquant 1992:136) notes that "one could say that I am in a sense hyperdeterminist."

Consequently, Bourdieu awards epistemological priority to objective conditions over subjectivist understanding (Wacquant 1992:11), even though he regards both as important. What this implies for the structure-agency debate is the dominance of structure over the habitus mind-set from which perceptions and behavioral choices are derived. This suggests that the selection of a course of social action is affected by life chances to a much greater extent than allowed by Weber or Giddens. Bourdieu's work indicates that life choices are not only constrained but actually shaped by life chances. Although individuals choose their lifestyles, they do not do so with complete free will as the habitus predisposes them toward certain choices. They have the option to reject or modify these choices, but Bourdieu maintains that an agent's choices are generally consistent with his or her habitus. Choices also tend to reflect class position because persons in a similar social class share the same general habitus. As Bourdieu (1990) explains, internalization of the same structures and common schemes of perception and appreciation produce the same or similar set of distinctive signs or tests: the result is a wide sharing of a class-based worldview. The habitus ("a structured and structuring structure") is structured by an individual's class conditions and, in turn, structures social action thereby reproducing class differences.

When it comes to lifestyles, Bourdieu (1984:171) says that they are operationalized as follows: (1) objective conditions of existence combine with positions in the social structure to (2) produce the habitus which consists of (3) a system of schemes generating classifiable practices and works and (4) a system of schemes of perception and appreciation (taste) that together produce (5) specific classifiable practices and works which (6) result in a lifestyle.

Lifestyle practices consist of particular forms of dress, food selection, music, art, sport, leisure activities, and the like—all of which express class, gender, and ethnic distinctions. Although lifestyles, including health lifestyles, can spread across class, gender, and ethnic boundaries, they typically originate in or are distinctive to a particular status group (Cockerham, Kunz, and Lueschen 1988). As Bourdieu (1984:172) explains, lifestyles are systematic products of habitus which, perceived in their relations to the schemes of habitus, become sign systems that are socially distinct. Lifestyles therefore function as forms of cultural capital with symbolic values. In Bourdieu's view the human body constitutes physical capital which is transformed into cultural capital as a consequence of social practices (Shilling 1993; Turner 1992). For example, different classes have different styles of exercising, eating, and dressing which define their bodies in particular ways. According to Australian sociologist Bryan Turner (1992:88), "weight lifting articulates working-class bodies, while jogging and tennis produce a body which is more at ease in the middle-class milieu or habitus." Thus, Turner (1992:90) concludes that the body is a site on which the cultural practices of the various social classes are inscribed.

It is therefore certain that structure is the dominant aspect of Bourdieu's concept of lifestyles. The notion of "structure" suggests persistence, repetition, and self-maintenance; hence, habitation, or the tendency of lifestyles to become habitual, is a key feature of his perspective. Lifestyles not only reflect social differences in ways of living but reproduce them. Compared to Weber and Giddens, whose ideas emphasize the voluntary nature of lifestyles, Bourdieu's approach is grounded on the social parameters of lifestyle selection. For instance, class-based lifestyles, as unitary sets of tastes or distinctive preferences, are practices that are classified and supported not only by participants within a class but also by other classes (Münch 1993). In sum, Bourdieu's contributions to our understanding of lifestyles fall into two major areas: (1) identifying the role of habitus in creating and reproducing lifestyles, and (2) emphasizing this role by showing how structure—or in Weberian terms, life chances—determines lifestyle choices. The gap between life chances and life choices in Weber's original analysis is significantly reduced through Bourdieu's concept of habitus which incorporates both within a single entity. The importance of Bourdieu's perspective is that it presents a theoretical model of social practice which includes consideration of the powerful effects of structure (Jenkins 1992). His work serves as an important counterweight to perspectives that view lifestyle decisions almost entirely in terms of personal choice and reflexive control (Williams 1995:601).

LIFESTYLES AND POSTMODERN CHANGE

The next step in conceptualizing the role of lifestyles in contemporary society is to consider the influence of postmodern social change on everyday life. In a historical sense, postmodernity refers to the social and political epoch that follows the modern era (Ritzer 1997). While there is considerable disagreement about the exact nature and definition of post-modernity, a common theme is that of an epochal shift, discontinuity, or break with modernity bringing new social conditions and principles with it (Baudrillard 1988; Best and Kellner 1991; Featherstone 1991; Smart 1993). There are three basic responses to this assertion: (1) claiming that a rupture has already occurred with modernity and we are living in a totally new era, requiring new concepts and theories; (2) denying that such a rupture has taken place by noting the continuities between the past and present; and (3) arguing for a dialectic of continuity and dis-continuity, theorizing about change from and continuity with modernity (Best and Kellner 1991:277–8). Unfortunately, no postmodern theorist to date has identified the exact point of rupture between modernity and postmodernity, possibly influencing skeptical scholars like Giddens to distinctly avoid the use of the term "postmodernity" and opt instead for a concept of "high modernity," signifying we remain in a late modern period.

Notions of an absolute break between postmodernity and modernity are unconvincing at present (Best and Kellner 1991). But so are denials of any rupture because it seems clear that a dialectic interchange between the present modernity and a new oncoming modernity is tak-ing place. For example, American sociologist Charles Lemert (1993) observes that something "real" is indeed happening with respect to post-modernity. In an admittedly speculative proposal, Lemert suggests that the modern era may have ended in 1979–80, between the high-energy periods of 1968 (student revolt against authority in the West) and 1989–91 (collapse of communism in the former Soviet Union and Eastern Europe). Social changes like the breakup of the Soviet bloc, the muliticulturalization of Europe and North America, the rise of cultural and sexual politics, changing patterns of social stratification and mobil-ity, and the emergence of a new world order do mean an era has ended and the effects on people's lives are real.

Although Lemert may or may not be correct about 1979–91 as the defining moment of postmodernism, his view that contemporary society is moving out of a postindustrial stage is supported by a number of sources (Baudrillard 1988; Bauman 1992; Beck 1992; Beck, Giddens, and Lash 1994; Best and Kellner 1991; Crook, Pakulski, and Waters 1992; Denzin 1991; Esping-Anderson 1993; Featherstone 1991; Harvey 1989; Jameson 1991; Lash 1990; Meštrovic 1991, 1992; Seidman 1994; Seidman and Wagner 1992; Smart 1992, 1993; Therborn 1995; Turner 1990). It is therefore apparent that something new is going on in the world and society is in a period of change in which it is beginning to experience the next era of social conditions. Consistent with this idea, British sociologist Barry Smart (1993:39) offers a good explanation of postmodernity by saying: "The idea of postmodernity indicates a modification or change in the way(s) in which we experience and relate to modern thought, modern conditions, and modern forms of life, in short to modernity." Smart suggests that since modernity itself is in a continuous state of flux and perpetually in motion, postmodernity is focused on transformations in society, culture, economics, technology, communications, and politics. While postmodernity has other meanings in other contexts and disciplines, much of its sociological relevance lies in its depiction of the destabilization of accepted meanings and efforts to adjust to new realities in society after industrialization.

The destabilizing effects of the new modernity caused radical change in the West and, as will be discussed at the end of this chapter, were terminal for the East. In the West, postmodern social change promoted multicultural and multiethnic societies; greater gender equality; increasingly rigid class boundaries, as it became more difficult to get into the upper class and out of the lower class; the rise of greater (but incomplete) European unity with the advent of the European Union; the solidification of knowledge as a commodity in the marketplace; computerization and the establishment of computer networks exchanging information on a global basis; continuing technological creativity; the growing dominance of the service sector of the economy over manufacturing, especially in the area of analytic services that identify and/or solve problems or provide strategic planning; a decline and lessened trust in the traditional industrial-age authority of politicians, physicians, lawyers, and other professionals; and greater individualization as people find themselves more on their own in a rapidly changing society.

According to German sociologist Ulrich Beck (1992, 1994), many of society's traditional ties and relationships have been weakened or lost. Family structures are being altered in the face of high divorce rates and increases in single-person and single-parent households. Peer group and work associations have also become weaker. And the greater the freedom for the individual, the greater the personal responsibility for his or her own welfare. While welfare states provide a minimal safety net to secure food and shelter for the impoverished, Beck explains that people generally have to bear responsibility for the consequences of their mistakes and that security can no longer be fully realized in society's "small" divisions (i.e., family and community). This development implies increasingly closer connections of individuals with the state in order to obtain health care, pensions, justice, civil rights, and financial support in surviving poverty.

Furthermore, Beck (1994:14) points out that even individualization is not a free decision of individuals. Individualization, in his view, is the need to invent new certainties for oneself and others lacking them in the face of the disintegration of the old certainties of industrial society. In this context, individualization is essentially an effort to design, manufacture, and stage one's own biography and the various commitments and social networks associated with it, such as educational certificates, career, marriage, and family life, in line with the conditions and models of the welfare state. As Beck concludes, individualization means that the standard biography becomes the chosen biography for most people.

The work of Swiss sociologist Marlis Buchmann (1989) suggests that this is indeed the case. She observes that with individuals being provided more benefits by the state, ties to the larger society are created and links to the family and community are lessened. Buchmann (1989:184–5) explains it this way: "As individuals participate in markets, enter the political sphere as citizens, and become recipients of welfare, obligations to social collectivities . . . such as the family, local communities, or status groups gradually vanish and render social identifications and identity constructions based on memberships in these collectivities increasingly obsolete." As people have to rely ultimately on the state to take care of them with respect to pensions, medical care, or unemployment subsidies, it is therefore not surprising that individuals have a more direct connection to the state than they did in past historical periods. The trend suggested by Buchmann's research is that social life is becoming more individualistic; however, she reminds us that the state—through its bureaucratic orientation and greater intervention in daily life—tends to structure the individual life course according to universal, rational principles of law. Consequently, increased state intervention counters individualism in late modern society. Buchmann (1989:185) states:

Thus, the more the individual life course is state-regulated (e.g., through age-grading and bureaucratically defined status allocation and status linkages), the higher its formalization and standardization. The simultaneously increasing individualization and standardization of the life course with the development of modern society engenders a peculiar dynamic: Life is less constrained by traditions and customs and thus more susceptible to individualized action orientations; these potential individual choices, however, must be made within the context of standardized and bureaucratized life patterns.

The implication consistent with the theme of this chapter is that individuals have greater choices and options than perhaps ever before, but these choices have boundaries. For example, the continuing destabilization of industrial-era norms, values, and traditional centers of authority in a postmodern scenario suggests even greater diversity in lifestyle options. Besides gaining more variety, lifestyles may become mixed or unattached to specific status groups (Featherstone 1987). On one hand, postmodern conditions promote uncertainty and diversity in lifestyle choices; on the other hand they push people toward making some kind of choice. This situation suggests lifestyle choices, health or otherwise, could become exceedingly diverse. However, even though lifestyle options in postmodern circumstances may be varied, they provide structure and express self-identity. And, as the author and his colleagues (Cockerham et al. 1997) suggest, they also provide *relief* in a rapidly changing world by reducing complexity. That is, lifestyle choices can promote a sense of stability and belonging for an individual by providing an anchor for the person in a particular social constellation of style and activity. They can, in fact, reflect what Beck (1994) calls the standard biography as people choose lifestyles representing a socially approved or normative pattern of behavior applicable to their group or stratum.

In sum, postmodern theorists typically portray the future as a period of increasingly rapid social change resulting in the destabilization of accepted meanings and the requirement for individuals to adjust to new social realities. Terms like deconstruction, decentering, and dedifferentiation common in postmodern literature signify the fragmentation and dissolution of traditional social structures and authority systems associated with both the industrial and postindustrial ages. Given the macro- or societal-level changes supporting this development, individuals—as noted especially by Giddens—will likely find themselves with greater behavioral options and fewer structural constraints than in the past. Consequently, the lifestyle choices people make and the social processes that shape those choices are likely to be an increasingly important factor in the conduct of everyday life.

This situation promotes the study of lifestyles as a major area of sociological inquiry, and health lifestyles as a particularly significant lifestyle form. If people, under postmodernity, have a greater diversity of choices and options and are subject to weaker structural constraints, agency would therefore appear to be the dominant force in social living. However, if structure shapes choices and options both materially and perceptually, structure may in fact be dominant. As Bourdieu (Bourdieu and Wacquant 1992:183) puts it: "Autonomy does not come without the social conditions of autonomy and these conditions cannot be obtained on an individual basis." In order to realize lifestyle choices people must have the capacity (life chances) to operationalize those choices. This situation applies to health as well as to other aspects of daily life. The point is that both agency/structure and choice/chance are essential components of lifestyle selection, but chance provides the basis upon which choices are made and translated into behavior thereby suggesting that chance or structure plays a somewhat more important role.

APPLICATION TO HEALTH LIFESTYLES

The work of Weber, Giddens, and Bourdieu converges and diverges on several points to stimulate thinking about health lifestyles. All three associate lifestyles with social class. Weber is concerned with status, Giddens with self-identity, and Bourdieu with social distinctions and taste. None of them seriously considers alternative status dimensions like gender, age, race, and ethnicity, even though these are major lifestyle variables. Nor do any of them discuss health in relation to lifestyle, with the exception of Bourdieu's (1984) examination of class differences in food habits and sports participation. Yet the work of each theorist represents a fundamental contribution to conceptualizing contemporary health lifestyles. Weber helps us to understand that lifestyles result from the dialectical interplay of choice and chance. Giddens explains that structure is both enabling and constraining. Weber and Giddens favor choice in this arrangement, but Bourdieu strongly emphasizes chance because of the perceptual boundaries it applies to choice. Our discussion will therefore be organized along the choice/chance debate, and follow with a section on the relevance of status variables other than class.

Life Choices

The notion of choice in health lifestyles would appear to be a relatively easy variable to operationalize because common sense would dictate that a person choose health. Weber (1958), for one, equates wanting to be unhealthy with being as foolish as wanting to be poor. Yet making choices is not that simple. Not only do life chances constrain choices, but matters are complicated further by the evolving uncertain character of postmodern social change. For example, in the United States there is clear evidence of a major decline in the professional authority and status of physicians (Cockerham 1998; Hafferty and Light 1995). At the same time, there has been an increase in individual self-responsibility for health (Crawford 1984; Goldstein 1992). This is manifested in the growing recognition by the general public that (1) major diseases—like heart disease, cancer, stroke, and AIDS—cannot be cured by medical care; (2) certain lifestyle-related activities—smoking, unhealthy eating and drinking habits, lack of exercise, male homosexuality, and the sharing of needles for drug injections—can end life prematurely; and, (3) consequently, medical treatment is not the automatic answer to dealing with all health problems (Crawford 1984). Thus self-control over personal behavior that affects health becomes the only remaining option to the health-conscious individual.

Strategies on the part of individuals to have healthier lifestyles in Western societies have therefore gained in popularity, although participation appears greatest among the upper and upper-middle classes (Blaxter 1990; Cockerham 1998; Cockerham et al. 1988; d'Houtaud and Field 1984; Goldstein 1992; Herzlich and Pierret 1987). People in these higher social strata experience greater life chances and are likely to have acquired a stronger sense of control over life situations than individuals in the classes below them (Mirowsky and Ross 1989). A major outcome of these cumulative experiences and the perception derived from them is a greater expectation that planning and effort will bring the desired result. Lower-class persons, in contrast, may be less likely to expect that their efforts to maintain their health will succeed, and be passive or less active in maintaining a healthy lifestyle.

Yet it is clear from studies in some Western countries, namely France, the former West Germany, and the United States, that health lifestyles have spread throughout the class structure (Cockerham et al. 1988; Herzlich and Pierret 1987). While there are undoubtedly differences in the quality of participation, most people do something to take care of their health. German sociologists Ronald Hitzler and Elmar Koenen (1994) point out that in the past health was a given—that is, health was considered essentially a gift from God; a person either had it or did not. But this perspective seems to be changing. In contemporary, more secular times, health has become a task, achievement, or performance of responsible individuals. People are therefore expected to create health for themselves.

Following Giddens (1991), Hitzler and Koenen note that people today have no choice but to choose whether or not they want to be healthy because health requires activity. The question thus becomes how they deal with choice. Hitzler and Koenen (1994:457) suggest three possible outcomes: (1) copy an existing lifestyle connected to a particular pattern of consumerism and follow it, rather than make new choices all the time; (2) be unable to choose a lifestyle thereby indicating problems in organizing one's life; or (3) individuality itself becomes a lifestyle, as is the case when a person always has to show that he or she is different. Apparently, most people choose the first option—they copy an existing lifestyle and adopt it as their own. Therefore, with the twenty-first century at hand, health lifestyles have become an activity that individuals are supposed to choose in a normative sense. They may not do so, but the normative and commonsense expectation is that they will do something to protect their health.

Life Chances

Chance mitigates choice. As previously noted, life chances—depicted in Weberian terms—are predominantly socioeconomic. Therefore, some people obviously have greater chances for realizing their choices than others. Whereas it is possible that life chances can reduce choices to almost zero in extreme situations, Giddens (1991) claims that no culture eliminates choice altogether. Rather, he finds, as previously noted, that the poor make lifestyle decisions, even though they do so under conditions of severe material constraint. With respect to health lifestyles it would appear that most people engage in some type of health-advancing behavior regardless of their socioeconomic position, but different social classes are likely to pursue different avenues toward health in terms of quality, distinctiveness, and probabilities for success (Blaxter 1990; Cockerham 1998). Numerous studies worldwide attest to the fact that the upper and middle classes in advanced societies have the longest life expectancy and the most positive levels of health (Cockerham 1998; Evans 1994; Marmot et al. 1991; Wilkinson 1996). Despite some expansion of upper-middle-class health lifestyles into other status groups, class still makes a difference with respect to health and health behavior.

Of course, one might argue that the decision to smoke or not smoke cigarettes, for example, ultimately falls to the individual regardless of his or her life chances. However, there is little empirical evidence to suggest that the contemporary patterns of social behavior we refer to as lifestyles are merely a deliberate product of independent individuals. As Bourdieu (Bourdieu and Wacquant 1992) explains, without the social conditions of autonomy, individuals cannot be autonomous. It is the internalization of external structures in the habitus, including not just past experiences and socialization but a realization by the individual of his or her social and economic circumstances, that largely determine perceptions. This is why Bourdieu depicts the habitus as socialized subjectivity whose limits are set by society and embedded in individual perceptions of social reality. Thus, habitus reacts to situations in a generally coherent and systemic manner by typically following a principle of consistency.

All this suggests that chance is a somewhat stronger component of lifestyle than choice. Choice is needed to initiate lifestyle participation but, as discussed, chance, or structure, provides the parameters, both material and perceptual, which largely shape the choices made. Therefore, consistent with Bourdieu's emphasis on the importance of structure, any concept of health lifestyles needs to pay particular attention to chance. Life chances influence lifestyles in two major ways: through socioeconomic resources and through perceptional boundaries derived from socialization and experience in a particular social milieu.

The Missing Link: Alternative Statuses

The origin and utilization of the lifestyle concept in the twentieth century is concentrated in the social stratification literature. The relationship between lifestyles and other forms of status—like gender, age, race/ethnicity, religion, and sexual preference—have not been fully explored, along with other variables like peer relations and the influence of advertising and mass media campaigns. For many individuals the group from whom they feel pressure to choose a particular lifestyle has a narrower orientation than their social class (i.e., military officers, teen peer groups, lesbians, Orthodox Jews). Members of these groups adopt norms and behaviors which constitute a lifestyle and cannot be explained by class alone. Other variables, like age and gender, may in fact induce age-specific or gender-specific lifestyles that transcend class boundaries. Consequently, socioeconomic status cannot be considered the sole determinant of lifestyles.

This appears to be particularly true of health lifestyles. Numerous studies identify dietary, exercise, drinking, and smoking patterns characteristic of specific groups regardless of their class position (Cockerham 1998; Dean 1989; Polednak 1989; Ross and Bird 1994). Strong religiosity, for example, has been found to promote healthy lifestyle practices (Dwyer, Clarke, and Miller 1990). There is evidence also that people tend to take better care of their health as they grow older by showing more careful food selection, more relaxation, and either abstinence or reduced use of tobacco and alcohol (Cockerham et al. 1988; Lüschen et al. 1995). But exercise declines significantly at older ages causing one major health lifestyle activity to be largely curtailed over the life span.

As for gender, American sociologists Catherine Ross and Chloe Bird (1994) found that men are more likely than women to exercise strenuously and walk but also more likely to smoke and be overweight. Men are particularly at risk if their advantaged position in the marketplace (higher salaries and decision-making roles) is accompanied by smoking, a high-fat diet, and passive leisure-time activities. Other research shows that men also consume more alcohol, and that women are more careful about their diet (Cockerham et al. 1988; Dean 1989). Consequently, gender can be regarded as one of the most important causal factors in health lifestyle selection. Women generally take better care of their health than men, and this pattern is seen in lifestyle differences.

Polish sociologist Zygmunt Bauman (1992) and Anthony Giddens (1991) suggest that individual needs for autonomy and identity tend to be translated into a need to acquire, possess, and consume specific goods for their symbolic values. In this context, the body takes on symbolic value as well, thereby linking lifestyles not only with status but health (Shilling 1993). Yet it is also clear that any concept of health lifestyles needs to go beyond an emphasis on socioeconomic status and consider other status variables, especially age and gender, which influence health practices.

Conceptualizing Contemporary Health Lifestyles

In order to construct a concept of health lifestyles, an important question needs to be answered: "What is it explicitly that lifestyle concepts are supposed to measure?" Ultimately, measures of health lifestyles should distinguish between groups of people on the basis of health behaviors and attitudes. The term "lifestyle" implies complexity and structure but nevertheless infers a unity, a pattern, or integrated sets of behaviors. The appropriate strategy is to identify these integrated sets of behaviors in relation to the groups that practice and reproduce them.

The challenge for sociological theory is to not focus on either agency or structure exclusively, but to develop an integrated concept. One way to connect agency with structure is demonstrated by Giddens (1984) in his dialectical notion of the duality of structure. However, Giddens's (1991) view of lifestyles emphasizes the importance of the actor (i.e., self-identity), while the structural component, though recognized as important, remains relatively abstract. Whereas this "abstractness" is itself part of Giddens's diagnosis of the condition of self and society in late modernity, it tends to undervalue structure.

Bourdieu's (1984) notion of habitus offers another route to explaining group- or class-generated lifestyles and the stability of such lifestyles under differing circumstances and over time. But contrary to the focus on the actor supplied by Giddens, the actor remains abstract in Bourdieu's approach. The obvious next step would be to require a concept that provides equity to actor and structure. However, while the relationship between choice and chance remains dialectical, it does not necessarily follow that the relationship has to be equal. Bourdieu (1990) points out that while the link between habitus and praxis is neither mechanical nor deterministic, the habitus predisposes the individual toward certain behaviors by providing a cognitive map of normative options. The dispositions produced are typically compatible with the constraints imposed by the larger social order and other factors like age and gender which set the individual on a stable and consistent course of action. Bourdieu (Bourdieu and Wacquant 1992) explains that this process is not a case of pure rational choice because the choices made are not completely autonomous. People may have control over their choices, but not necessarily over the social and psychological conditions that underlie those choices.

It seems likely, in line with Bourdieu's perspective, that structure exercises a dominant role in structure-agency relations and lifestyle formation. In the author's view, Bourdieu's assertion that structure—as internalized by the habitus through socialization and experience—largely determines the perceptual boundaries underlying choice is correct. Not only does structure shape perception, it also provides the context for social interaction. Even Weber, despite his emphasis on choice observes that there are structural circumstances that can severely inhibit individual choice. For example, Weber (1958:54) referred to the capitalist economy as an "immense cosmos" which is presented to individuals as an "unalterable order of things." "It forces the individual," states Weber (1958:54), "in so far as he [or she] is involved in the system of market relationships, to conform to capitalistic rules of action." Therefore, when it comes to health lifestyles, choices involving health-related activities are to a large degree shaped by habitus and operate in a more or less routine manner in a person's life.

This consistency and routinization most likely prevail, even in postmodern conditions where people are detached from the certainties and modes of living of the industrial age and subjected to evolving social circumstances with greater behavioral options. People are confronted with an ever increasing body of health knowledge and invested by the larger social order with greater personal responsibility to live in a healthy manner. At the same time, they witness industrial traditions, including those of medical power, being weakened by postmodern change. This leaves individuals subject to choosing a health lifestyle in a situation of decreasing certainty and increasing complexity. Lifestyles are opportunity structures in that people adopt them for the gains they feel they can acquire which include both a material form to their self-identity and an anchor in a particular style of living. The latter, we would argue, promotes a sense of stability by reducing complexity in a rapidly changing social environment. Having met the pressure of having to choose a health lifestyle, they can pursue it in a more or less routine fashion along the lines set by their habitus.

While choices are made by individuals, they nevertheless fit into a structural scheme grounded in group behavior. This situation presents a methodological challenge, since many structural approaches that emphasize the effects of life chances on individuals tend to underestimate the creativity of social agents. Conversely, many microsociological approaches concentrate on the perspective of the social agent and tend to underestimate the interdependence of patterns of social behavior and life chances which produce the structure of lifestyles. To distinguish between phenomena with varying degrees of complexity it is necessary to focus on a number of variables that must be analyzed if the typical structure of a pattern of behavior is to be reproduced. This situation is made more complex by the variety of resources and behavioral options available to individuals within a postmodern setting. However, there is a lack of empirical evidence showing that health lifestyles are merely a deliberate product of "postmodern" individuals created independently of life chances. Lifestyles are grounded in life chances—which include socioeconomic status, age, gender, and race/ethnicity—and the social options those chances provide. The crucial point is that the choice-chance relationship must be conceptualized as a complex form of inter-action involving the interplay of the two.

The definition of health lifestyles as collective patterns of health-relat-ed behavior based on choices from options available to people according to their life chances reflects the dialectical choice-chance relationship. It incorporates the interplay of choice and chance along Weberian lines, but omits the requirement that choices are voluntary. The structure pro-vided by life chances may require particular choices be made, which ren-ders a voluntary process of decision-making difficult or impossible. A person in this circumstance would have to deal with whatever lifestyle paths are open, not some idealized and unavailable situation. Other indi-viduals might have a much greater range of choices in similar or differ-ent situations, but the fact remains that everyone's choices are con-strained (even though the constraints may be overcome) by the reality of their chances of realizing them. Therefore, Bourdieu's assertion that structure determines the perceptual boundaries underlying choice is persuasive when it comes to conceptualizing lifestyles in general and health lifestyles in particular. Individuals have the free will to choose, but their choices invariably have limits.

HEALTH LIFESTYLES AND SOCIALISM

It might be argued that the concept of health lifestyle is a particularly Western idea that is not relevant to the everyday experiences of people in the former socialist countries. Lacking a tradition for mass media public health campaigns, antismoking laws, and active counseling and follow-up by health care providers, it is not likely that former Soviet-bloc residents would adopt a healthy lifestyle as part of their general ori-entation to living. In the former Soviet Union, for example, physicians (who often smoked themselves) would advise their patients to smoke less harmful cigarettes with filters than give up smoking altogether (Specter 1995). Fresh fruits and vegetables were difficult to obtain in the winter, and leisure-time exercise was uncommon in a region lacking indoor facilities for year-round participation. Adding the tendency toward heavy drinking on the part of males, overall health-related lifestyles in this region were obviously more unhealthy than healthy.

The prevailing policy orientation under socialism was to invest the responsibility for health in the state rather than the individual. Secondary prevention of health problems requiring contact with physicians and early detection of disease was the norm; primary prevention in which individuals are encouraged to live a healthy lifestyle was not emphasized. In the West, individual responsibility for health was a major feature of public health policy. Western governments were criticized, however, for under-emphasizing the role of the state in fostering poor health in situations of poverty, unsafe workplaces, and poor enforcement of environmental protection laws. Thus, policy debates in the West were focused primarily on the state's role in providing a healthy environment and standard of living, along with greater responsibility for financing and delivering quality health care. Individuals were nevertheless expected to pursue a healthy lifestyle and protect their own health as best they could.

In contrast, health lifestyles in the former socialist countries were not an issue of individual responsibility with the state expected to reinforce this effort. The state, in fact, assumed responsibility for health, and individuals were relegated to a more or less passive role in the provision of services. People were expected to go to doctors for preventive measures like checkups and immunizations, and to receive care when they were sick. They were not generally expected to participate in a lifestyle that would maintain or improve their health. This does not mean, however, that individuals did not have a health-related lifestyle. Everyone has a lifestyle, including a health lifestyle. But in the East, those lifestyles, as noted, promoted poor health. The main causes were structural, and improvement was not simply a case of the individual changing his or her behavior. An ineffective health policy, societal-level stress resulting from a failing economic and political system, and especially the regionwide evolution of an unhealthy lifestyle, principally among middle-aged males, constituted a social condition that—in the absence of individual responsibility for health—ended lives prematurely.

Furthermore, it should not be expected that the introduction of a capitalist system into a previously socialist one would manifest itself in the same manner as in Western models. As American sociologist Neil

Smelser (1997) explains, the notably headlong rush to a market system met resistance from forces influenced by the past communist and social-ist traditions of those countries. "We thus observe," states Smelser (1997:83), "the apparently contradictory results of favoring wage labor, the profit system, and the consumer economy but at the same time favoring socialist-type guarantees (mainly in the form of welfare) that reduce the risks and inequalities that have always been built into mar-ket capitalism." Smelser suggests that there is not much doubt about which set of forces will ultimately prevail (capitalism), but at present the ambivalence and struggle between the two opposing systems of market capitalism and former communism continue.

Thus, a major adjustment to new, postmodern conditions in the former socialist countries revolves around the issue of personal welfare. Bauman (1992) refers to the former socialist countries as "patronage states." "Under the rule of the patronage state," comments Bauman (1992:163), "freedom of individual choice in all its dimensions was to be permanent-ly and severely curtailed, yet in exchange the less prepossessing aspects of freedom—like individual responsibility for personal survival, success, and failure—were to be spared." In other words, the state provided for the individual and his or her needs, while the individual in turn abandoned self-reliance and personal freedom on behalf of the omnipotent state. To many, observes Bauman, the state was a shelter. Education and health care were free, while old-age pensions and low-cost housing and food, along with guaranteed employment, were state benefits. The removal of the state's welfare safety net and the burdening of the individual with respon-sibility was a mixed blessing. For some—especially elderly pensioners and people in late middle age who had lived exclusively under communist rule and had supported, as well as believed in, the former system—the end of communism was particularly traumatic.

Health lifestyles in societies providing high levels of patronage and dis-couraging individual initiative in most aspects of daily life are not likely to feature a strong sense of individual responsibility. Such lifestyles would not be expected to be in line with the philosophy of the state, and under socialism an emphasis on healthy living on the part of the individual was absent. Nor was this sense of responsibility likely to appear quickly in the aftermath of communism's fall, when alternative state mechanisms of sup-port were not readily available and norms for maintaining one's own health were still lacking. It is therefore not surprising that mortality rates have increased, not declined, in most former Soviet-bloc countries during the early transition to capitalism. Whereas personal choices concerning health were limited under socialism, most people did not have the means to avail themselves of the increased options that appeared with the fledgling market economy. In a very real sense, life chances were still overpowering choices. And, as will be seen in subsequent chapters, chance, or the structural component of health lifestyle, explains the downturn in life expectancy in the region better than any other single factor.

A final question that needs to be considered is related to the origins of lifestyles in general and health lifestyles in particular. Lifestyles do not just happen by themselves; rather, they are constructed by people pursuing similar ways of living over time which evolve into a pattern of behavior. This behavior is characteristic of specific groups, social classes, and societies, and the individuals within them. Historical traditions, culture, social values and tastes, levels of education, political philosophies, group and class orientations, and especially socioeconomic conditions all contribute to lifestyle formation. Therefore, when it comes to health and other lifestyles, the psychology of the individual alone is not the sole determining factor. Lifestyles also have their inception in structural conditions external to the individual, and are reflections of the social structural entities out of which they evolve. This means that efforts to change health lifestyles in the former socialist countries will require changes at the macro as well as the micro level. In the United States, for example, there have been several important macro-level measures that have promoted individual self-protective behavior. Perhaps the most significant ones to date have been the ban on smoking in public places and the legal requirement of seatbelt use in automobiles (Sweat and Denison 1995). In the former Soviet bloc the problem of unhealthy living patterns developed out of poor-quality socioeconomic conditions and a lack of encouragement for individuals to take personal responsibility for their own health. Consequently, as will be discussed in future chapters, in order to transform the pattern of health lifestyles it will be necessary for these countries to adopt macro-level changes that will encourage and reinforce any forthcoming efforts of individuals to promote their own health.

Chapter 4

Russia: Life Expectancy and Social Change

As the hub of communist power and site of the steepest decline in life expectancy, Russia represents a special situation among the former socialist countries. What happened in Russia is key to understanding what happened throughout the Soviet bloc because the Russian system of socialism was dominant in the region. This chapter discusses Russia's health profile over the course of the late nineteenth century to the present. Chapter 5 covers the country's current health crisis.

In examining Russia's health situation, it is important to recognize that there is a distinct pattern of health problems corresponding to each stage of a country's change in social organization from a rural to an urban society and from an agricultural to an industrial economy. The principal causes of death in rural agrarian societies are infectious and parasitic diseases, which typically result in high infant mortality and relatively low life expectancy. Once urbanization and industrialization are underway the pattern changes. Life expectancy increases, infant mortality declines, and infectious and parasitic diseases are generally curtailed, but heart disease, cancer, and other chronic illnesses emerge as the leading causes of death. Applying this pattern to the Russian experience since the late 1890s will help locate the point at which the country's development diverged into a pathway toward increased mortality.

This chapter was written with the assistance of Vladimir M. Shkolnikov, Ph.D., Head, Laboratory for Analysis and Prognosis of Mortality, Center of Demography and Human Ecology, Russian Academy of Sciences, Moscow.

THE LATE IMPERIAL PERIOD

In 1897, Russia was a rural agrarian society ruled by an autocratic monarch, Czar Nicholas II, whose family had governed since 1613. The overwhelming majority (86%) of the Russian Empire's population of 125 million people lived in the countryside. The nobility typically had estates in the country as well as houses in town. Much of Russia's art, literature, music, and ideas about political and social reform were associated with intellectuals—such as Alexander Pushkin, Leo Tolstoy, and Ivan Turgenev—who either lived on or frequented country estates (Roosevelt 1995). At the opposite end of the social spectrum in estate life were the peasants who provided the labor. Some homes of the nobility on the estates were lavish and others were not, but the houses of peasants were almost universally simple, small, dark, dank, smelly, smoky, and crowded (Pipes 1995; Suny 1998; Tian-Shanskaia 1993). American historian Priscilla Roosevelt (1995) describes the estates as "two kingdoms"—one consisting of the landowner and his or her dependents, guests, and domestic servants, and the other of farmers, craftsmen, and artisans living in villages. "In his own kingdom," states Roosevelt (1995:220), "the landowner was sole ruler, but in certain dealings with the other kingdom (for example, in collecting the state tax on all adult males, sending recruits to the army, making his serfs work on road maintenance, and maintaining order) he was also acting as the czar's agent."

According to a 1858–59 register of Russian nobility, approximately 1 million people belonged to the nobility. However, after excluding certain groups of nobles (Russians with nonhereditary titles, Poles, and other foreigners), only an estimated 274,000 persons qualified as the hereditary Russian nobility (Pipes 1995). And, of the latter, only some 1,000 families were extremely wealthy. Many of the remainder were not so fortunate, despite their social rank. The hereditary landed nobility, especially those from affluent families, were the dominant class by a wide margin in Russian society. As Ronald Suny (1998:12) observes: "Their very way of life—their wealth, style, behavior, and distance from ordinary people, all of which stemmed from their birth—gave them a sense of their own right to rule and to be obeyed."

As for the middle class, it was small and insignificant. British historian Richard Pipes (1995:191) refers to this class in its imperial Russian version as the "missing bourgeoisie." Little money was in circulation, Russia was outside of Europe's principal trade routes, and the country produced few entrepreneurial merchants and industrialists. Russia's early industrialization was financed by the state and there was some success in this area in the late nineteenth century with respect to mining, iron and steel works, and textile production. This development produced a small but growing working class of industrial laborers, composed mainly of former peasants, who resided in a few important urban centers. As Suny (1998:24) points out, "Russia's first industrial revolution, in the 1880s and 1890s, was a mammoth change for the agricultural empire, but it stopped short of transforming the whole of Russian society."

The bulk of the population in 1897 (about 85%) were peasants, the majority of whom could not read or write. Until emancipation in 1861, they had been serfs—a de facto form of personal slavery. Serfs in Russia and Eastern Europe were legally bound to the land they farmed and could be transferred with it to a new landowner. The landed gentry provided loans, protection, and the administration of justice; in return, the serfs worked a certain number of days in the landlord's fields. On other days they farmed plots assigned for their own use. Serfs could not leave their estate, marry, or learn a trade without the landowner's permission. Emancipation, however, allowed them to receive parcels of land to work as their own, with the legal title to the property held by their village. The landowners in turn were compensated by the government for the land they turned over to the peasants. Most peasants, however, continued to live in disadvantaged circumstances even though by 1916 they owned some two-thirds of the cultivated land in European Russia (Pipes 1995). They had been granted long-term government loans to pay for the property, which added significantly to their financial debt. As Pipes (1995:167) explains:

> The combined pressure of excessive fiscal burdens, social and economic disabilities and an uncontrollable population growth created a situation which made it increasingly difficult for the Russian peasant to support himself from agriculture. In 1900, it was estimated, he covered only between a quarter and a half of his needs from farming; the remainder he had to make up in some other way. The solution readiest at hand was to hire himself out to landlords or rich peasants as a laborer, or else to lease land and till it either on a sharecrop basis or in return for various services; in the latter event, he reverted to the status of a semi-serf.

Table 4.1

Life Expectancy at Birth in Russia, 1896–1996

Year	Males	Female
1896	30.9	33.0
1910	—	—
1926	39.3	44.8
1938	40.4	46.7
1958	61.9	69.2
1965	64.0	72.1
1970	63.0	73.4
1980	61.4	73.0
1984	61.7	73.0
1985	62.7	73.3
1986	64.8	74.3
1987	64.9	74.3
1988	64.6	74.3
1989	64.2	74.6
1990	63.8	74.4
1991	63.5	74.3
1992	62.0	73.8
1993	59.0	72.0
1994	57.5	71.0
1995	58.2	71.7
1996	59.7	72.5

SOURCES: Shkolnikov 1995, 1997; State Committee of the Russian Federation on Statistics 1996.

Whereas emancipation did not appreciably improve the socioeconomic position of most peasants, it also seriously eroded the position of the nobility. Many of the landed gentry could not maintain their style of estate life without the income produced by serf labor, and were forced to sell their landholdings. As a class, the nobility lost most of its economic foundation in the final decades of the empire's existence and their political influence correspondingly declined (Pipes 1995). According to Orlando Figes (1996:47):

> The Emancipation came as a rude shock not just to the economy but also to the whole provincial civilization of the gentry. Deprived of their serfs, most of the landed nobles went into terminal decline. Very few were able to

respond to the new challenge of the commercial world in which as farmers—and less often industrialists and merchants—they were henceforth obliged to survive. The whole of the period between 1861 and 1917 could be presented as the slow death of the old agrarian elite upon which the czarist system had always relied.

It is not surprising, given the social conditions of the time and the country's rudimentary health care system, that life expectancy was relatively short. As noted in chapter 2, nearly half of all Russian infants in the 1880s failed to live until age five because of diarrhea and respiratory diseases (Tian-Shanskaia 1993); cholera, typhus, and tuberculosis also took the lives of many children and adults (Figes 1996). Infant mortality as late as 1913 was particularly high by European standards, at 245 infant deaths per every 1,000 births. According to table 4.1, Russian males lived an average of only 30.9 years and females 33 years in 1896. In contrast, French males and females lived about 15 years longer at that same time, with an average of 45.4 years for men and 48.7 years for women.

THE SOVIET PERIOD

The revolution of February 1917 destroyed the Russian Empire. In the face of social unrest, military defeats, and an underdeveloped economy unable to meet wartime or civilian demands, the czar had refused to seriously consider reforms or end participation in World War I. The huge government bureaucracy remained inefficient; nationalism and a desire for independence were surfacing in the non-Russian parts of the empire; disastrous military campaigns and huge casualties from fighting continued; while war-weariness and widespread loss of confidence in the regime promoted a strong desire for change (Figes 1996). As Polish sociologist Piotr Sztompka (1993:301) points out, revolutions are the most spectacular manifestations of social change and mark fundamental ruptures in a country's historical process, while reshaping its society from within. This is exactly what happened as the Russian Empire, jolted into a new form through revolution, emerged as the Soviet Union.

Suny (1998) suggests that the history of the Soviet Union can be viewed as the tale of three revolutions, each identified with a single individual. The first revolution is that of 1917, which Vladimir Lenin used to establish the Soviet state; the second was Joseph Stalin's program to create a socialist society and economic system in the 1930s; and the third was Mikhail Gorbachev's "revolution from above" in 1985–91, which attempted to dismantle the Stalinist heritage. This third revolution ended in the collapse of the Soviet Union.

Victory by the communists in their October 1917 armed takeover of power from the provisional government and in the subsequent civil war gave Lenin the opportunity to recreate Russian society. The nobility was destroyed as a social class. As previously noted, many Russian nobles, including the czar and his immediate family, were killed. The majority of the survivors fled abroad, while others were imprisoned or managed to remain and live quietly in social circumstances far below their previous station in life (Massie 1995; Radzinsky 1992). Some social control features of the former czarist system were retained, such as an authoritarian style of government, a secret police, and labor camps for dissidents. The role of religion in public life was ended as the state became not only secular but overtly antireligious. When it came to social stratification, the break with the past was complete, and a radically different social order came into existence in the 1920s emphasizing upward social mobility for workers and peasants.

The new Soviet class structure was a state-engineered system of social stratification organized around a one-party dictatorship, a centrally planned economy, and a growing military-industrial complex (Rigby 1990). This structure was shaped by Stalin and was continued and even strengthened after his death. The major organizing principle in the beginning was coercion, but after Stalin material incentives and privileges became more important (Zaslavsky 1995). The central government, through its role as a patronage state, became a mechanism for redistributing the nation's wealth, with priority given to leading persons in the Communist Party. According to Russian sociologist Aleksei Kochetov (1993), the class structure of Soviet society by the mid-1980s featured the party elite—the *nomenklatura*—as the most powerful and privileged group. As shown in table 4.2, the *nomenklatura* was composed of less than 1% (0.7%) of the population and had access to the best goods and services available to Soviet society. Members of the party elite had special privileges with respect to medical care, housing, consumer goods, vacations, travel abroad, and schools to help their children perform well on the examinations for admission to higher education. Suny (1998) reports that during the Brezhnev era these appointed officials were guaranteed long tenure in office. Freed from close control, they often exercised arbitrary power and engaged in extralegal and corrupt practices that brought them material gain. "Accountable to their superiors rather than their constituents," states Suny (1998:435), "this conservative, entrenched, well-educated and privileged group of top party officials and regional [party bosses] made up a separate upper class of privilege and power."

Table 4.2

The Class Structure of Late Soviet Society

Class	Percent
Nomenklatura	0.7
Administrators and managers	3.5
Literary and artistic intelligentsia	1.8
Technical specialists	18.8
Low-skilled clerical/technical workers	5.0
Industrial workers	41.3
Service workers	13.0
Peasants and agricultural workers	15.0
Unclassified	0.9
Total	100.0

SOURCE: Adapted from Kochetov 1993.

Next in the social hierarchy, constituting 3.5% of Soviet society, were top administrators and managers of important state agencies and key industries. In Western terms, this group might be viewed as the upper-middle class. Below them was what could be considered the Soviet middle class, namely the literary and artistic intelligentsia (1.8%) and technical specialists (18.8%). The latter, many of whom were employed as skilled industrial workers, engineers, and scientists in the military, nuclear, and space sectors, represented the bulk of the middle class. They served as symbols of success for the social strata below them (Zaslavsky 1995). The next occupational group, as shown in table 4.2, were low-skilled clerical/technical workers (5%), followed by the largest single category in the Soviet class structure of industrial (blue-collar) workers (41.3%). Service workers (13%) and peasants and agricultural workers (15%) were at the bottom of society. Although peasants remained at the lowest rung of the social ladder as in czarist times, the size of this class had shrunk considerably from 85 to 15% of the total population.

What is sometimes forgotten in the aftermath of the revolution and the civil war, followed by Stalin's purges, police state repression, the drive toward industrialization, and forced movement of peasants into a collective farm system, is that many Soviet citizens were enthusiastic about building a new society. "In the 1920s," states American historian Walter Laqueur (1994:8), "Soviet power rested on the presence of hundreds of thousands—perhaps millions—of enthusiasts, mainly young, whose imagination had been fired by the [communist] vision." The Communist Party promised not only good government and a viable economy but also social equality and justice for all. The need to rebuild the country, defeat Nazism, and achieve superpower status was a cohesive factor in Soviet life. "The careers of members of the new elite quite apart," comments Laqueur (1994:13), "there was a feeling among young Communist enthusiasts that the collective was infinitely more important than the individual." If regimentation and loss of personal freedom were the price to pay for forging a socialist society, many people seemed willing to do it. According to Fred Coleman (1996:124):

> The Soviet economic system was not always a top-to-bottom failure, of course. In the beginning of Stalin's rule, from the late 1920s to the early 1940s, his rigid command economy made eminent sense, as the U.S.S.R. surged ahead from a primitive agricultural backwater to a modern industrial society at breakneck speed. Only the iron fist could put order in Russia's chaotic house so rapidly.

However, as Coleman observes, once the Soviet Union was in the ranks of the developed nations, the command system of centralized planning for industrial production could not keep pace with the West. "The functioning of the command economy," states Spanish sociologist Manuel Castells (1998:31), "was based on the fulfillment of the plan, not on the improvement of either products or processes." Soviet specialists in all fields lacked the freedom to innovate and make decisions on their own. They had quotas and directions from above and were discouraged from going beyond boundaries set by Communist Party bureaucrats. The entire economy was managed by a hierarchy of committees headed by the state planning commission (Gosplan) which in turn took its orders from the Communist Party through the central government's council of ministers. By all accounts the Soviet Union missed the revolution in information technologies that occurred in the mid-1970s (Castells 1998). The flow of free and uncensored information was incompatible with the communist system. At a time when there was a critical shift in computer capabilities in advanced capitalist countries, the Soviets were unable to integrate the rapid diffusion of the new information technologies into their controlled system. "In short," states Coleman (1996:124), "forced to choose between progress and control, the Communists chose control." Even in the workplace, Party control remained the top priority over job performance and effectiveness. Coleman (1996:124) found that:

> Among other things, Party overlords decided which projects specialists could undertake and on what terms. They also limited the funding granted specialists, computer time, and access to Western scholarship to the point where relatively few Soviet economists, scientists, technicians, and other specialists ever lived up to their potential. In addition, Party loyalty rather than proven ability in a field of specialization determined promotion and success. In the end, the Soviet Communist Party educated some of the world's best scientists and technicians, with the potential to raise the economy to new heights, then largely wasted them for political reasons.

Despite the millions of deaths from revolution, war, famine, and Stalin's mass executions, health and life expectancy began to improve in the Soviet Union in the 1920s and 1930s. As discussed in earlier chapters, an army of health care workers was mobilized, trained, and distributed throughout the country in a successful effort to lower infant mortality and eradicate infectious diseases. As shown in table 4.1, by 1926, life expectancy for the Soviet Union's Russian male population had improved to 39.3 years and for the female population to 44.8 years; by 1938, there was a slight increase to 40.4 years for men and 46.7 years for women. However, the greatest increase in longevity took place between 1938 and 1965, as the average Russian male reached 64 years and female 72.1 years in life expectancy. These figures, however, include only the population under the system of civil registration. The low life expectancy of Siberian labor camp inmates was not counted.

The 1950s and early 1960s were a period of even more significant economic growth, scientific achievement, and global military power for the Soviet Union. Inequality in income between social classes was considerably less than in the West because of state-controlled salaries. There was almost complete job security, housing was cheap, and hunger was not a problem for most people. Moreover, the country had become a largely urban society by the 1960s, as people moved to the cities to enjoy a higher standard of living—even with government restrictions on internal migration. Yet the overall standard of living remained far below that of the West and, in some instances, even below that of Eastern European countries, like East Germany and Czechoslovakia. Housing was gradually improved so that, by 1975, over 70% of urban families no longer had to share their apartment or a bathroom with other people, but these dwellings nevertheless remained cramped and shortages of housing persisted. The average diet was heavy in carbohydrates—especially from bread and potatoes—and the consumption of meat, fresh fruit, and vegetables was significantly lower than in the West. In shopping for food and other consumer items, Soviet citizens often spent 2–3 hours daily waiting in line. And, as previously noted, the quality of health care available to the general public was lower than in the West.

The high point of Soviet development was reached in the mid-1960s about the time Leonid Brezhnev (1964–82) replaced the ousted Nikita Khrushchev (1953–64) as premier and Communist Party leader. Although some facets of Soviet life, such as wages and housing, improved in the early Brezhnev years, the general strategy of Soviet leaders toward domestic affairs under Brezhnev was maintenance of the status quo. The Brezhnev era generally is known as a period of economic stagnation in which the *nomenklatura* consolidated their privileged position and discouraged change. At the same time, industrial and agricultural problems were seriously undermining the country's economic well-being. By the early 1970s, industrial performance slowed as worker productivity lagged, money-losing state enterprises were kept open, and investment remained concentrated in heavy industry and weapons production. According to Castells (1998:21), "perhaps the most devastating weakness of the Soviet economy was precisely what was the strength of the Soviet state: an over-extended military-industrial complex and an unsustainable defense budget." Profits from oil and gas revenues helped offset losses in manufacturing for some time, but this measure only forestalled economic decline. Agricultural production was also unsatisfactory as the nation's collective and state farm system was unable to produce and deliver enough food to feed the country. As Coleman (1996:1370) explains:

> Here is how the Soviet planned economy worked on agriculture: farmers got paid the same whether they loaded their trucks fully with produce or not. Often they didn't. The trucks then went to the nearest railway station,where more problems arose. Because of the country's poor road system, most foodstuffs reached the distant cities by rail. But industrial goods had the priority on freight train shipments. So fresh food often rotted at the railhead, waiting for empty freight cars. Food that went out on trains in time often spoiled later in poor processing or storage plants. In the end, Soviet authorities themselves estimated that between the farm and the

family dinner table, some 40% of the country's food supply got ruined by poor transport, processing, and storage facilities.

Beginning in 1965, life expectancy for Russian men entered a period of long-term decline. Table 4.1 shows that in 1970 Russian males lived 63 years on average, down 1 full year from 1965. Russian females, in comparison, saw their life expectancy increase 1.3 years (from 72.1 years in 1965 to 73.4 years in 1970) during the same time frame. By 1980, male life expectancy had declined further to 61.4 years, followed by a very slight recovery to 61.7 years by 1984. Life expectancy also fell slightly for females to 73 years between 1970 and 1984.

Why did life expectancy turn downward in 1965? The best explanation seems to be that Russia had reached a point in its modernization when an important epidemiological change had taken place: infectious diseases had been brought under control and chronic illnesses associated with aging had become dominant. By the mid-1960s, the accumulated effects of a generally unhealthy male lifestyle in the post–World War II period—involving high levels of alcohol consumption and smoking, poor diet, and little exercise—had triggered an epidemic of heart disease among susceptible middle-aged males. The Soviet health care delivery system, oriented toward dealing with infectious diseases, was ill-prepared and unfocused on coping with chronic illnesses. There is a relatively inexpensive and universal approach to treating communicable diseases, namely vaccination for prevention and antibiotics for treatment. Chronic disorders, like heart disease and cancer, however, are considerably more expensive to treat and require an individual approach to patients, which often involves a modification of their lifestyle. But this approach was not compatible with communist values, which emphasized the welfare of the collective over the individual. Under Brezhnev, the collective orientation to patient care was not changed, more medical resources were not provided, nor was Soviet medicine redirected toward shifting its focus. The health care delivery system, like the economy in general, was not reformed, and it stagnated under a "business as usual" mentality. This approach failed when confronted with the increasing incidence of heart disease.

Not only was life expectancy decreasing in the Soviet Union but the economy was continuing to worsen as well. Economic and political reform was desperately needed. Unexpectedly, change came in the form of a revolution from the Soviet leadership. On 10 March 1985, the elderly and ailing Soviet premier Konstantin Chernenko died after only 13 months in office. The previous premier, Yuri Andropov, had been in office less than 16 months before dying of cancer. Both of these leaders had spent much of their time as head of state in hospitals. As a result, there was finally some support in the Soviet Union's ruling body, the 10-man Politburo, for the appointment of a younger person. The older Politburo members had a candidate from their age-group and the majority of votes to elect him, but adroit political maneuvering by 54-year-old Mikhail Gorbachev brought him the premiership on 11 March. Calling the decisive meeting shortly after Chernenko's death, when three members of the opposition were too far away from Moscow to return in time, Gorbachev got the votes he needed (a majority of 4 to 3) to become premier. The outmaneuvered opponents had no alternative but to accept the decision and show unity to the outside world.

Gorbachev served for only 6 years (1985–91), but, as Coleman (1996) points out, he accomplished more than any other statesman in the world during the last half of the twentieth century. While most foreigners believe he changed the world for the better, many Russians feel he changed their country for the worse (Coleman 1996; Keep 1995; Remnick 1993; Roxburgh 1992; Suny 1998). When he took office, the Soviet economy was failing and increasingly unable to produce both modern weapons and consumer goods in the cold war competition with the West; agricultural production continued to be disappointing; and, moreover, the armed forces were bogged down in an unpopular war in Afghanistan. Gorbachev's time in power was in effect a revolution from above in that he instituted radical changes that turned the Soviet Union from a one-party communist state with a parliament that did what it was told, into a country with a fledgling multiparty political system that provided a variety of candidates for election to office. Censorship was replaced by freedom of the press after a difficult struggle, police-state repression was removed, foreign travel was authorized for the general population, and efforts were made to introduce a limited free-market economy. The Soviet Union also ended its political and economic isolation in order to become more fully integrated into the world community. Steep cuts were made in its military forces, and Soviet troops were withdrawn from Afghanistan without securing victory. Finally, Gorbachev made it possible for East and West Germany to be reunited and for the other countries of Eastern Europe to follow an independent course in managing their domestic and foreign affairs.

However, at home he was increasingly criticized because the Soviet Union's standard of living continued to decline and the country's status as a superpower was ending. Although Gorbachev was a genuine reformer, his reforms had not gone far enough. He changed the political system but still wanted a major role for the Communist Party; he tried to move the economy in the direction of capitalism, but was uncomfortable with private ownership of property and set limits on profits; and he wanted to keep the various nationalities in the Soviet Union together, despite their strong desire for independence. His vision seemed to stop short of the measures needed to complete the revolution. His changes angered the conservative, hard-line communists who were losing power, but did not go far enough to satisfy the reformers.

In an effort at compromise, Gorbachev placed hard-line communists in several important government positions. It was this group, including his vice president, that led a military coup against him in August 1991. While on vacation at his villa near the Black Sea, Gorbachev was confined in his compound by security forces after he refused to step down from the presidency. In the meantime, Boris Yeltsin, the Russian head of state, led opposition to the coup in Moscow. Climbing up on top of a tank, Yeltsin spoke to a large crowd, denouncing the coup and calling for civil disobedience and labor strikes. Army units sent to enforce the state of emergency joined Yeltsin instead. Some 200,000 Muscovites demonstrated in the streets and many surrounded Yeltsin's headquarters at the Russian parliament to prevent an attack. In the face of this massive display of opposition the coup's leaders lost their nerve and some flew to Gorbachev's villa to ask forgiveness. They were arrested, and the coup collapsed. Above all, the coup failed because of popular resistance to it (Roxburgh 1992:214).

On his return to Moscow, however, Gorbachev missed an opportunity to reinstate himself as the leader of reform. Instead, he talked about reforming the Communist Party so that it could be the force behind *perestroika*, or restructuring. But, as British journalist Angus Roxburgh comments, ordinary people in Moscow showed what they thought of that by toppling statues of communist leaders and demanding an end to the party itself. "No longer," states Roxburgh (1992:216), "would his term *perestroika* apply to what was happening: this was a real revolution, sweeping away the Communist Party, its system, its values, its statues, and its leaders." It took Gorbachev several hours to realize this—a delay that inflicted permanent damage on his position. Too late, he gave up leadership of the Party and ordered it to close its offices.

The collapse of the Communist Party was followed by the breakup of the Soviet Union into 12 independent states. The three Baltic republics of Latvia, Lithuania, and Estonia declared themselves independent countries outside of this new organization. Gorbachev soon found himself out of power as a private citizen, while Yeltsin became president of Russia. Gorbachev had begun the revolution but Yeltsin, who understood the mood of the people better, carried it to its conclusion.

There is no evidence to suggest that health care was a priority under Gorbachev. He did not increase funding for health services, nor even discuss health matters in his memoirs (Gorbachev 1996). His main contribution was to revitalize an anti-alcohol campaign which was primarily intended to improve worker productivity and decrease alcohol-related absenteeism (Holmes 1997). But the effect of this campaign on life expectancy during its short duration (1984–87) was dramatic (Shkolnikov and Nemtsov 1994). Again, referring to table 4.1, in 1984—the first year of reduced production and consumption of alcohol—male life expectancy had a slightly higher level of 61.7 years compared to 61.4 years in 1980. The next year, 1985, with Gorbachev in power and seriously cracking down on alcohol use, Russian male longevity rose to 62.7 years, followed by 64.8 years in 1986 and 64.9 years—an all-time high—in 1987. In 1988, the highly unpopular campaign was ended and male life expectancy dropped to 64.6 years. At the conclusion of Gorbachev's tenure in office male life expectancy had fallen back to its 1960s level of 63.5 years. Female life expectancy, in turn, rose from 73 years in 1984 to 74.6 years—also an all-time high—in 1989; however, a slight decline set in for 1990–91, and the figure stood at 74.3 years at the end of the Gorbachev era.

THE POSTCOMMUNIST PERIOD

From 1991 to the present, the Russian Federation had to struggle with massive changes in the wake of the Soviet Union's demise. Constructing a new society and economic system in the aftermath of 74 years of entrenched communism has been exceedingly difficult. Substitute institutions to replace the ones in the former system had to be created. There was no practical experience with capitalism, and manufacturers and distributors did not initially know how to produce, market, and sell goods in such a system (Goldman 1996). Customer-oriented services were practically unknown. Nor was there an existing legal system of codes and laws to support commercial activities. Moreover, the notion of formal contracts and individual entrepreneurship for personal gain is unfamiliar in Russian tradition. Many Russians, especially peasants, express a cultural hostility to elite groups, private interests, and profit-making (McDaniel 1996; Pipes 1995; Schmemann 1997).

The central government's budget has also been adversely affected by its significant shortfalls in tax collection. Some Russian companies elude taxes by conducting much of their business in the form of barter, such as a furniture company trading finished products for raw materials, Western currency, food and holiday facilities for workers, places in kindergartens for workers' children, and hard-to-get supplies (Burawoy and Krotov 1992). Many companies have simply refused to pay taxes in a system in which tax dodging has become an art (Gordon 1997). And, to make matters worse, Russia's mafia became extremely powerful once communist control ended. In the absence of strong legal and police safeguards, many businesses secured protection from either the mafia or lawful private protection services. The mafia, in turn, expanded from criminal enterprises into legitimate businesses and, in many instances, became a de facto government of its own—so great is its current power (Goldman 1996).

But there are also some successes. Many large formerly state-owned enterprises were transferred to private ownership (although they were often acquired by their former managers using insider knowledge and personal relationships); private shops, stores, and companies were opened; foreign investment grew; both imports and exports increased; and there was a virtual boom in protection services for security and in the construction business to meet the demand for refurbished and new offices and personal dwellings. Some progress was also made in business law, while government efforts to improve tax codes and collection procedures are underway. Furthermore, inflation has slowed and in the late 1990s the Russian economy finally showed improvement after its chaotic downward slide in the aftermath of communism's collapse. Industrial production rose 1.9% in 1997, after declining every year since the late 1980s, and the nation's gross domestic product grew 0.4% after years of decreases. However, in 1998 the Russian economy imploded, destroying their gains. The failure to collect taxes was a key factor in the collapse, along with a decline in oil revenues. The Russian government was unable to pay its bills and the equivalent of billions of dollars were lost as banks and businesses failed, the stock market crashed, inflation soared, and the ruble was officially devalued. Rising prices, unpaid wages and salary cutbacks, and layoffs continued as the government sought an end to the crisis. Although most long-range prognostications about Russia's future are positive, it is the short term that is highly problematic (Åslund 1995; Remnick 1997).

Russia is also experiencing the third transformation of its class structure during this century. The exact form of the new class system has not yet emerged, but the upper class will likely consist of the most successful capitalist entrepreneurs and leading government officials. Some members of the old elite have, as noted, converted their former bureaucratic privileges into economic wealth by becoming private owners of former state enterprises. However, with the end of socialism and the decline in influence of many former communist bosses, a new elite of reform-oriented capitalists and their allies in government has emerged. It is this new elite that is grasping power, although some former communists have attempted to slow reform and continue socialism where possible. Their opposition has included political dissent and armed revolt, as seen in a failed attempt to seize power from Yeltsin's central government by a counterrevolution in Moscow in 1993.

About 3 to 5% of the population has become wealthy. However, this group faces varying degrees of resentment from the general population because of the widespread belief they acquired their fortunes either through illegal activities or by taking advantage of their previous positions (Brym 1996). There is a very wide gap in income between this stratum and the remainder of Russian society. As Canadian sociologist Robert Brym (1996) points out, in 1991 the richest 10% of all Russians earned 4.5 times more than the poorest 10%; by 1994, the ratio had jumped to 15 times more, making Russia one of the most inegalitarian countries in the world with respect to income.

Russia has a small but increasing middle class and a large working class but, in contrast to Soviet times, the lower class is expanding due to the growing ranks of the unemployed from obsolete industries, along with the elderly trying to survive on inadequate pensions, unskilled laborers, and peasants. The latter are claiming they cannot adopt private farming because they do not have the livestock and machinery they need, nor the money to purchase them; they also are unsure about how to divide the land between themselves or even how to work on their own (Schmemann 1997). Consequently, only some 5% of Russia's agricultural landholdings are family-owned farms.

For the majority of Russians life has become particularly hard since the end of the Soviet Union. Estimates of the proportion of people living below the poverty line in 1998 stood at over one-third of all Russians (44 million of Russian's 148 million people). The discontent stems not only from unemployment—which was 8% of the workforce in 1997 and even higher in 1998—but also from the growing impoverishment of those with jobs, as prices rise and salaries stay low. State-controlled salaries and pensions in particular remain at low levels and are sometimes not paid for weeks at a time. Physicians, intellectuals, and artists especially have been subject to pauperization within the middle class (Boutenko and Razlogov 1997). Some feel, in the absence of state support, that their government has abandoned them and yearn for the economic stability and better living conditions provided by state dependency under communism (Brym 1996). However, there is neither a widespread desire for a return to communism, nor an adoption of militant nationalism (Remnick 1997). Rather, among many people, there is an ambivalence featuring nostalgia for the czarist period, offset by a feeling that this era was unavoidably doomed; a dislike of communism for ruining the country, but pride in its achievements; and satisfaction about communism's fall countered by fears of uncertainty about the future and the potential of a dictatorship (Schmemann 1997). The overall mood in the new Russia is perhaps captured best by Pulitzer Prize–winning American journalist David Remnick (1997:ix–x) who writes:

> To live in Moscow at century's end is to exist in a strange and contradictory landscape, one filled with both ruin and possibility. The signs of a fallen totalitarian state persist; Lenin gazing out over October Square; the apartment buildings on Leninsky Prospekt built by prisoners of the Gulag; the old and poor marching on May Day, sometimes even carrying portraits of Stalin. At the same time, the newspapers (when they are not shilling for the government at election time) are alive with real news and reflect varied commentary; stores with high-quality goods are opening all over; the airports are mobbed with people traveling abroad as often as their income will allow. On Lubyanka Square, the statue of the founder of the secret police, Feliks Dzerzhinsky, is gone (it was torn down after the collapse of the August [1991] coup); and, nearby, a stone from Soloviki, the first of Lenin's concentration camps, honors the millions killed under the old regime. And yet the old KGB structures (using new names and old methods) are still at work. All around, the bright lights of commerce flare while the mayor orders police to arrest the homeless and put them on trains.
>
> In the provinces, the contrasts are more subtle, but they are there all the same: Japanese businessmen eating in the sushi bars of Khabarovsk while laborers in town wait six months or more for their wages; in Ivanovo, where three quarters of the workforce has been laid off from the textile mills, television carries up-to-the-minute reports from the film festival at Cannes; the scholars and scientists of Novosibirsk arrive home after yet

another conference at Harvard and walk past refugees living in the airport; the shoppers in Murmansk try to read the labels on bottles of Norwegian shampoo and try not to worry too much about the nuclear waste threatening their city, their harbor; on the Leningrad Highway, a new Mercedes with dark-tinted windows streaks past a beggar. The symbols of transformation are stark and banal and true. But the transformation of Russia is not merely a matter of its outward signs—its relics and innovations. The process rolls in the mind and heart of every Russian. Although the epochal new stories are now a matter of history—the end of the Cold War, the end of communism, the end of empire—every Russian (even the young) lives in multiple worlds: in a past that still shapes his thinking and language and habits; in the sometimes unbearable present, with its economic and psychological shocks; and in the future, which is even more unknowable, more unpredictable, than it is elsewhere.

During this period of transition, it is not surprising that already poor health conditions worsened. The overall quality of life for many people declined even further, the health care delivery system deteriorated even more and poor health lifestyles, as seen in the continued abuse of alcohol and cigarettes, along with high-fat diets and lack of exercise, were epidemic. As shown in table 4.1, life expectancy for males fell from 63.5 years in 1991 to a modern low point of 57.5 years in 1994. However, male longevity improved to 58.2 years in 1995 and again to 59.7 years in 1996. Yet it is entirely too early to determine whether male life expectancy has actually improved or simply that the most unhealthy middle-aged men have already died thereby boosting current longevity figures. Female life expectancy also fell after the collapse of the Soviet Union, dropping from 74.3 years in 1991 to 71 years in 1994. Women registered a slight improvement to 72.5 years in 1996.

CONCLUSION

It is clear from the above discussion that the present state of Russian longevity is linked to the social, economic, and political conditions prevalent in the country since the mid-1960s. As economic indicators and living standards have fallen, so has length of life. The most recent postcommunist period has seen a particularly steep decline in the health of the population as a result of the acceleration of a long-term downward trend. Chapter 5 reviews the current state of the Russian health crisis.

Russia: The Current Health Crisis

The most severe rise in peacetime mortality in a developed nation in modern times has taken place in Russia. The purpose of this chapter is to determine whether or not the nation's health crisis has passed, and to examine the contributions of policy, societal stress, and health lifestyles to the current situation.

HAS THE CRISIS PASSED?

The research reviewed in previous chapters shows that the decline in life expectancy in the former Soviet Union began in the mid-1960s and was primarily fueled by rising mortality among middle-aged men with working-class backgrounds. This appears to still be the case, although the most recent data on life expectancy show a slight increase for males in 1995 and 1996, and for females in 1996. Does this mean the health crisis has passed and Russia is returning to a consistent upward trend in life expectancy? First, it needs to be realized that Russia's devastating demographic problems have not come to an end. Russia's mortality rate in 1994 was 15.7 deaths per 1,000 persons; the rate improved in 1995 to 15 deaths per 1,000, but this still is one of the highest mortality rates in Europe and Asia. Furthermore, the birth rate has declined from 23.2 births per 1,000 persons in 1960 to 9.3 per 1,000 in 1995. Overall,

This chapter was written with the assistance of Vladimir M. Shkolnikov, Ph.D., Head, Laboratory for Analysis and Prognosis of Mortality, Center of Demography and Human Ecology, Russian Academy of Sciences, Moscow.

Russia had 840,000 more deaths than births in 1995, resulting in a natural population decrease of 5.7 per 1,000 persons.

The Russians have not been producing enough newborns to replace every deceased individual since before World War II, but this has not been an unusual trend in developed countries as women entered the labor market in large numbers and started exercising greater choice over how many children to have. Consequently, birthrates have also fallen in Japan and the West, including dropping below replacement levels in Germany and Italy. Yet, between 1990 and 1995 the number of children born in Russia was 3.7 million fewer than between 1985 and 1990. With the death rate accelerating in the 1990s, the population of Russia is now shrinking at a much faster pace than in any of the other former Soviet republics, with the possible exception of Latvia and the Ukraine. It is also shrinking at a faster rate than in the former socialist countries or any other developed nation showing a population decline. If current trends continue, the population of Russia could decrease by over 30 million people over the next 50 years. This would be a demographic disaster for Russia's future workforce.

The male life expectancy of 59.7 years in 1996 may represent an important upturn from the 1994 figure of 57.5 years. Yet, any claim that life expectancy is rising is offset by the notion of an accumulation effect. There is a limit to the number of middle-aged men with cardiovascular disease, and life expectancy may have risen because the most susceptible of these men have already died. Thus, the "accumulated" effect of these deaths over time may have left behind a smaller but longer-living cohort, which is not the same as the general male population living longer. This might have especially been the case in the aftermath of the Soviet Union's demise, when male life expectancy plunged downward in the face of rising mortality. For example, the mortality rate for Russian men age 40 to 49 in 1990, one year before the end of the Soviet Union, was 9.2 deaths per 1,000; in 1995, the rate had jumped to 16.3—an increase of 77%. Additional data are needed over the next several years before it can be conclusively determined that male life expectancy is actually on the rise.

The major causes of death also provide insight into the state of Russia's health crisis. Table 5.1 shows death rates from major causes per 100,000 persons in Russia between 1990 and 1995. Mortality from all causes rose from 1,116.7 deaths in 1990 to a high of 1,566.1 in 1994, then dropped to 1,496.4 in 1995. The same pattern is seen in table 5.1 for deaths from cardiovascular disease, which rose from 617.4 per 100,000 in 1990 to 837.3 in 1994, with a decline to 790.1 in 1995. Accidents, poisonings, and injuries, which have a strong relationship to alcohol use, are the second leading killer and follow the same pattern, as do respiratory diseases. Cancer rates remained relatively stable, but digestive diseases—which include cirrhosis of the liver—increased from 28.7 deaths per 100,000 in 1990 to 46.1 in 1995, while infectious and parasitic diseases rose from 12.1 to 20.7 over the same period.

Table 5.1

Major Causes of Death per 100,000 Population, Russia, 1990–1995

Causes of Death	1990	1991	1992	1993	1994	1995
All causes	1,116.7	1,137.5	1,215.6	1,446.4	1,566.1	1,496.4
Cardiovascular diseases	617.4	620.0	646.0	768.9	837.3	790.1
Accidents, poisonings, and injuries	133.7	142.2	173.0	227.9	250.7	236.6
Cancer	194.0	197.5	201.8	206.9	206.6	202.8
Respiratory diseases	59.3	55.7	57.9	74.5	80.8	73.9
Digestive system diseases	28.7	28.9	32.8	38.3	44.1	46.1
Infectious and parasitic diseases	12.1	12.0	13.1	17.3	20.1	20.7
Other diseases	71.5	81.2	91.0	112.6	126.5	126.2

SOURCE: State Committee of the Russian Federation on Statistics 1996.

The consistent rise in deaths from infectious and parasitic diseases is troubling because such diseases are generally preventable and have been largely eradicated in developed countries. Fear of poor-quality vaccines and the potential of infection from dirty needles are among the reasons fewer children have been inoculated in recent years. Although the over-all number of deaths from infectious diseases remains relatively small in comparison to mortality from heart disease, the incidence of diphtheria, typhoid, and tuberculosis significantly increased in the 1990s. This development signifies worsening, not improving, economic and social conditions and a deteriorating health care delivery system.

Another related problem is the major rise in sexually transmitted diseases. In 1996, some 10 million Russians were reported to have a sexually transmitted disease (Specter 1997b). In 1990 the rate for syphilis was only 6 cases per 100,000 persons. In 1996 there were 217 syphilis cases per 100,000—which is 50 times greater than in the United States and Europe. Where there is a spread of syphilis and other sexually transmitted diseases, AIDS cannot be far behind. And, indeed, HIV infections have been increasing, largely through the sharing of contaminated needles in narcotic use. The city of Kaliningrad (formerly Königsberg when it was part of Germany), a Russian enclave between Poland and Lithuania, has the highest proportion of HIV-infected people in Europe—about 1,850 cases out of a total population of 400,000 in 1997. While AIDS is less common in cities deeper in Russia, the possibility of its spread in cities like Moscow, Saint Petersburg, and elsewhere is enormous, given the fact that practically no AIDS education and prevention programs exist and little money is available to initiate them (Specter 1997b, 1997c). The AIDS virus has entered Russian society at a time when drug abuse is spreading among young people, which creates the potential for the disease to spread as well.

The Russian health crisis, therefore, is far from being over. Serious health problems remain and new ones, like AIDS, are appearing on the horizon to threaten the health and life span of the population. In order to better assess Russia's health prognosis, next I examine the role of the three primary social determinants of life expectancy in the former socialist countries—policy, societal stress, and health lifestyles—in their Russian context.

POLICY

The major focus of health policy in postcommunist Russia has been to bring the nation's severe health problems under control and create a health insurance system. Funding for health care declined from 3.3% of the GDP in 1990 to 1.8% in 1993 (Boutenko and Razlogov 1997), and stood at 2.2% in 1997. Taking into account that the GDP has decreased by 35 to 40% since the end of the Soviet Union, the real purchasing power of the funds allocated to health has fallen drastically. The financial condition of the country handicaps the Yeltsin government from providing more money and, if more funding was forthcoming, much of it would likely be wasted in Russia's sprawling, cumbersome, and repetitive health care system (Specter 1998). For example, in the city of

Tomsk there are 88 hospitals for 500,000 residents—more than in Boston. According to Michael Specter (1998), 12 hospitals treat only tuberculosis patients—including 1 exclusively for children with a staff of 134, a school, and several buildings—but never treated more than 20 patients at any one time in 1997. Few children had the disease. Hospitals in Russia still receive their budget from the central government based on their number of beds, regardless of how many of these beds are needed or even used (Sheiman 1994). It is not surprising, accordingly, that Russia has more hospital beds per person than any major country in the world (130 beds per 10,000 people, compared to the United States with over 35 beds per 10,000). Both the municipal and university medical centers in Tomsk also offer basically the same services, while there are 2 large heart centers and 4 cancer centers. Despite obvious duplication of many types of care, little has changed in the organization of health care delivery in Tomsk under the Russian Federation. Essentially, the old Soviet system remains intact in that city and throughout Russia, even though reforms are being planned or implemented.

Except for facilities that have been privatized, the ownership and operation of clinics and hospitals remain the responsibility of the Ministry of Health. Management duties are delegated from the Ministry of Health to subordinate agencies in the Russian Federation's administrative areas, and down to local neighborhoods and rural sections. Most of the population receives health care at polyclinics located in cities or in rural health centers. Polyclinics are paid by the government on the basis of the potential number of visits and the size of their staff; physicians are paid a salary by the state, which in 1995 was about $145 a month. A particular health practitioner is responsible for a designated number of people. A physician who provides primary care, for instance, would be assigned about 2,000 people on the basis of their residency. Patients are free to select their own physician if they are willing to pay out of pocket; otherwise, they utilize the physicians to whom they are assigned. People who can afford to pay for health care have access to the best doctors and hospitals available; they also typically receive faster and higher-quality services.

In 1991 and 1993 Russia passed legislation establishing a new system of health insurance, consisting of compulsory and voluntary plans (Curtis, Petukhova, and Taket 1995; McKeehan 1995; Sheiman 1994). The compulsory health insurance plans are financed by central government subsidies for pensioners and the unemployed, along with contributions (3.6% of payrolls) from employers to cover workers. This coverage is compulsory for all employees, provides the same basic benefits without choice, and is administered by local government agencies. The voluntary private insurance plans, which anyone can purchase out of their own pocket, provide supplemental benefits. The intent is to move away from the former Soviet method of paying for health care directly out of the central government's budget and to replace it with a universal system of health insurance providing basic benefits for all participants. At present, this new system is in its infancy and has not been fully established. The administrative structure needed to collect payroll taxes, process claims, and make payments to providers has been slow to develop because of a lack of experience and money (Light 1992). Furthermore, the process of collecting employer contributions has been difficult because many business enterprises have gone bankrupt, are in serious difficulty, or have avoided paying taxes (Lassey, Lassey, and Jinks 1997). This effort at reform, nevertheless, marks a major change in financing health care for the Russian people, although the results are far from complete.

The current system of health care in Russia has seen only limited successes. The diphtheria epidemic which swept across Russia between 1993 and 1997 was curtailed, as was an influenza epidemic in 1995. A principal goal of the health care delivery system, initiated in Soviet times, has been to reduce infant mortality. Table 5.2 shows that infant mortality has traditionally been lower in urban than in rural areas, which is a typical worldwide pattern. For the total population, infant mortality decreased from 36.6 deaths per 1,000 live births in 1960 to 17.4 in 1990. After the collapse of the Soviet Union, infant mortality rose from 17.8 deaths per 1,000 births in 1991 to 19.9 in 1993, but this increase was largely due to changes in registration procedures. In 1995 the infant mortality rate was 18.1; preliminary figures for 1996, not shown in table 5.2, are 17.4 per 1,000, the same rate as 1990. Basically, there have been no significant changes in the infant mortality rate since the 1970s (Boutenko and Razlogov 1997).

With respect to the current health crisis, Russian policy efforts have brought little change to date. The former Soviet system is still in place and the widespread prevalence of heart disease among middle-aged males remains unchecked. Government funding continues to be below minimum levels and fiscal reform, including health insurance, is incomplete. From a policy standpoint, it does not appear that the crisis has passed, nor have policy measures yet been effective. Many Russians, in fact, feel that their health care system has deteriorated even further since the end of the Soviet period and are particularly concerned about emergency care and hospital conditions (Brown and Rusinova 1997).

Table 5.2

Infant Mortality Rate for Urban, Rural, and Total Populations of Russia, per 1,000 Live Births, 1960–1995

Year	Urban	Rural	Total
1960	34.9	38.1	36.6
1965	26.4	26.7	26.6
1970	22.1	24.5	23.0
1980	21.2	24.0	22.1
1985	19.8	22.8	20.7
1990	17.0	18.3	17.4
1991	17.2	19.1	17.8
1992	17.6	19.1	18.0
1993	19.2	21.4	19.9
1994	18.0	19.5	18.6
1995	17.4	19.8	18.1

SOURCES: Shkolinkov 1997; State Committee of the Russian Federation on Statistics 1996.

SOCIETAL STRESS

It is impossible to deny the fact that the current period of adjustment after the demise of the Soviet Union has been highly stressful for the Russian population. There is a notion of "shock" mortality, which implies that the rapid and negative effects of the collapse of communism stimulated an increase in death rates. While it is true that the population has been stressed and mortality from natural causes has risen during the postcommunist period, it is not clear how the "shock" of the transition contributed to the death toll. Unfortunately, studies of stress-induced mortality in Russia are lacking, and without empirical data it is not possible to gauge the direct psychological effects of stress in this situation. Furthermore, when it comes to the effects of macro-level stress on the health and longevity of a large population, it is difficult, if not impossible, to measure the relationship. In a broad sense, large-scale societal process-es, specifically those of economic change, can be correlated with health outcomes, like a general rise or fall in mortality from heart disease or in admissions to mental hospitals (Brenner 1973, 1987; Turner, Wheaton, and Lloyd 1995). But making the connection is not that simple. It is very difficult to substantiate a precise cause-and-effect relationship between a major social event, like an economic depression or the downfall of communism, and the health of any one individual, because of the potential for a wide range of variables intervening in the individual's situation and modifying the stress outcome. Possible intervening variables include personality, social support, genetic background, social class, and upbringing. For instance, research on the effects of social support (feelings of being loved, accepted, cared for, and needed by others) on persons subjected to unemployment, stressful everyday life events, occupational difficulties, homelessness, and natural disasters like tornadoes and floods, shows that social support can act as a buffer against the adverse effects of stress (Cockerham 1996, 1998; Mirowsky and Ross 1989; Thoits 1995). Social support is typically obtained within families and from positive relationships with friends, religious worship, and activities with local groups and clubs. The evidence is overwhelming that people with the strongest level of social support have fewer health problems.

Variables like social support, the hardiness of one's personality and sense of coherence, class position, and the like help account for the fact that while some people are overcome by stress in given situations, others are not. Nevertheless, it is apparent that social and economic conditions beyond the direct control or influence of the average person can create stressful circumstances that force people to respond to them. For vulnerable individuals, the stressful circumstances may promote poor health. In the Russian situation, the strongest stressor appears to be the loss of security as the social benefits of communism (guaranteed jobs and price controls) disappeared and low wages and pensions made life extremely difficult in the face of the increasing cost of living. Stress may have been most severe for middle-aged working-class males tasked with being their family's main provider. Despite the official policy of gender equality in the former Soviet Union and the large-scale movement of women into employment outside the home, men still opted for the dominant role in gender relations (Gray 1990). For example, communist propaganda from the very beginning supported equality between the sexes but idealized male productive labor as the major source of material wealth in society and the basis for constructing the future socialist order (Weitz 1996). Images of leadership and strength were invested primarily in men. As American historian Eric Weitz (1996:316–17) points out:

[Communist] political art, drawing upon both social and traditional Russian representations, depicted the blacksmith as the ideal proletarian—the powerful man forming the steel of socialist construction and imbued with near-magical powers. Occasionally he has a female helper, but certainly not a female fellow blacksmith. His male comrades, wherever they are—the Soviet Union, Germany, France, Italy—are invariably strong, determined, and skillful. They gaze upward, heroically, into the socialist future, concentrate deeply on their labor, or march together shoulder to shoulder.

Weitz finds that no image of femininity dominates communist representations in the way that the heroic and combative male provides a uniform and consistent model of masculinity. Communist images of women blended female activities in building socialism, participating in athletics, and working on the job, with the general societal role of females in homemaking, child-rearing, and supporting the heroic socialist husband. The communist man was supposed to be masculine and dominantly strong, regardless of gender equality. Thus, the change from socialism may have been more distressing psychologically for men than women if they were unable to provide for their families. On the other hand, because of the convergence of men and women in the labor force under socialism, both sexes would have been equally exposed to the same macro-level stress from the transition to postcommunism. Women workers would have faced job insecurity, layoffs, and loss of income like the men. Research from the Czech Republic suggests that the stress of men and women workers was about the same during the economic reforms in that country (Hraba et al. 1996). Whether there was a similar outcome in Russia is not known, but it is clear that both sexes experienced the same stressful societal conditions.

Moreover, there are ample accounts of Soviet men failing to help in the home or be particularly supportive of their wives. Women worked at their jobs and then did nearly all the shopping, cooking, housework, and child-rearing (Buckley 1997; Gray 1990). Life may in fact have been more difficult for women, who carried most of the burden in family affairs besides a full-time job outside the home. Yet the fact remains that men are the major victims of the shortened life expectancy that arose during the Soviet period and increased during the postcommunist era. If women were highly stressed, this situation did not produce the massive casualties from heart disease and alcohol-related problems that occurred in males. In the absence of relevant studies, it may be conjectured that the greatest effect of societal stress was in promoting an unhealthy male lifestyle through excessive drinking and smoking, rather than in causing a direct physiological "shock" leading to the heart attacks that women generally escaped. But regardless of the mechanisms through which stress operates, life in Russian society has remained difficult, even though the initial psychological distress associated with the transition out of communism seems to be over.

HEALTH LIFESTYLES

Since unhealthy lifestyles were identified as the primary social determinant of the decline in longevity in the former socialist countries, it is necessary to identify the specific components of these lifestyles to further understand their contribution to the current health situation in Russia. In conceptualizing a particular Russian lifestyle that promotes a shortened lifespan, two variables—gender and age—are immediately recognized as significant on the basis of prior discussions. As already noted, the downturn in Russian life expectancy has had its greatest impact on the middle-aged male population. When women have been affected, it has been middle-aged women who have shown the greatest increase in early mortality. Following the collapse of the Soviet Union, when life expectancy declined for both men and women, male sex and middle age remained the most powerful predictors of rising mortality.

The best evidence in this regard comes from the work of Vladimir Shkolnikov (1996). As shown in figure 5.1, Shkolnikov compares the ratios of age-specific death rates in Russia for the years 1991 through 1994 with those in the year 1987. In 1987, when Gorbachev's anti-alcohol campaign ended, longevity for Russian men was at its highest point ever (64.9 years) and at one of its highest for women (74.3 years). Overall, figure 5.1 shows that the increase in middle-aged mortality, which had been interrupted by the anti-alcohol campaign, was reestablished in the early 1990s. The largest relative increases in age-specific mortality rates occurred for men ages 25 to 44 and women ages 15 to 44. At younger and older ages the increases were much smaller. Although the patterns of mortality for the years 1991–92 and 1993–94 appear to be similar, there are two important differences: (1) in 1993–94, the levels of mortality are much higher; and (2) in 1993–94 there is a significant increase in mortality for people between 44 and 64 years of age. This means that while premature mortality remained primarily a middle-

age phenomenon, its highest levels were shifting into late middle age by
1993–94.

Figure 5.1

Ratios of Age-Specific Death Rates in 1991, 1992, 1993, and 1994 to
those in 1987.

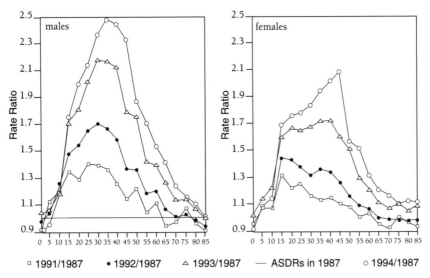

□ 1991/1987   • 1992/1987   △ 1993/1987   — ASDRs in 1987   ○ 1994/1987

SOURCE: V. M. Shkolnokov, "The Russian Health Crisis in Mortality Dimensions," Harvard
Center for Population and Development Studies, Working Paper Series No. 97.01, March
1997. Reprinted with permission.

Table 5.3 shows the age-specific contributions to the decreases in life
expectancy by gender for the years between 1991 and 1994. The greatest
concentration of mortality for males was in the 15–64 age-group, and the
contribution of late-middle-aged men (45–64 years) was increasing,
while that of younger men (15–44 years) was decreasing. For instance,
in 1991–92, 53.8% of the total decline in life expectancy was caused by
an increase in mortality at ages 15 to 44 and 40% by the increase at ages
45 to 64; in 1992–93, the proportions for the two age-groups were
roughly equal at 41.1 and 42.1%, respectively; but, by 1993–94, the
15–44 age-group was responsible for 34.2% of the rise in mortality, while
the 45–64 age-group was responsible for 53.1%. Although women show
a significantly lower contribution to increased mortality than men, they
show a similar pattern with respect to age.

One of the possible reasons why women live longer, even in times of stressful social and economic transition, is the fact that females are biologically stronger at birth, as seen in the greater prevalence of disease and physiological problems among male babies (Cockerham 1998). The female hormone estrogen also plays a protective role for women against cardiovascular diseases prior to menopause. And particularly important is the fact that women generally take better care of their bodies. Current research shows that Russian women, in contrast to their male counterparts, drink much less alcohol, smoke fewer cigarettes, and eat a healthier diet (Bridger 1997; Hurt 1995; Leon et al. 1997; Palosuo 1997; Palosuo et al. 1995, 1998; Ryan 1995; Stack and Bankowski 1994).

Table 5.3

Age-Specific Contributions to Decreases in Life Expectancy at Birth: Russia, 1991–1994

	Males					
Age	1991–92	%	1992–93	%	1993–94	%
0–14	0.089	-6.0	-0.110	3.6	0.008	-0.6
15–44	-0.798	53.8	-1.258	41.1	-0.498	34.2
45–64	-0.593	40.0	-1.288	42.1	-0.774	53.1
65+	-0.180	12.2	-0.406	13.3	-0.194	13.3
Total	-1.482	100.0	-3.062	100.0	-1.458	100.0

	Females					
Age	1991–92	%	1992–93	%	1993–94	%
0–14	0.163	-30.6	-0.182	10.0	0.051	-6.1
15–44	-0.448	83.9	-0.400	22.1	-0.204	24.7
45–64	-0.355	66.4	-0.670	37.0	-0.436	52.7
65+	0.105	-19.7	-0.560	30.9	-0.238	28.7
Total	-0.535	100.0	-1.812	100.0	-0.827	100.0

SOURCE: Shkolnikov 1996.

The majority of studies on health lifestyles measure differences in alcohol use, smoking, leisure-time exercise, and diet, along with regular visits to physicians for routine physical examinations, automobile seatbelt use, personal appearance or hygiene, and relaxation (as a means for coping with stress). There is a paucity of data on physical exams, seatbelt use, personal hygiene, and relaxation in Russia, but enough research exists on the other, especially important, variables of alcohol and cigarette consumption, exercise, and food habits to help formulate a model of a Russian health lifestyle.

Alcohol Use

There is strong evidence to suggest that the single most important health lifestyle characteristic of Russians (especially males) is high alcohol use. In 1995, Russians consumed 4.1 gallons of hard liquor per capita—the highest in the world. To put this situation into perspective, Nemtsov and Shkolnikov (1994) point out that children under the age of 15 (who make up one-quarter of the population) are almost all nondrinkers, and adult women (who make up one-half of the population) consume only one-eighth to one-tenth of the amount consumed by men. Consequently, some 90% of all alcohol is consumed by one-quarter of the population: adult males. Each adult male averages about 160 to 180 half-liter bottles of vodka consumed a year, which comes to a bottle almost every other day. About half of all adult men and almost a third of the women suffer some physical consequence of long-term drinking; perhaps half of all deaths can be attributed at least partially to alcohol (Specter 1997a). Heavy alcohol consumption is responsible not only for the high rates of heart disease, but also for an upsurge in deaths from accidents, alcohol poisoning, and cirrhosis of the liver.

The most authoritative study of the relationship between drinking and life expectancy in Russia was conducted by Shkolnikov and Nemtsov (1994) who determined that excessive alcohol consumption was the single most important determinant of the increased mortality. They investigated alcohol production (both official and unofficial), sales, and reported and real consumption between 1971 and 1993, with a focus on the effects of Gorbachev's 1984–87 anti-alcohol campaign on mortality. Calculating the difference between observed and expected deaths by sex and age, Shkolnikov and Nemtsov found that longevity increased 3.2 years for males and 1.3 years for females during the campaign's duration, with the greatest advance in life expectancy taking place in 1986. It might seem surprising that a significant decline in alcohol consumption could reduce mortality rates from heart disease so directly, given the usual long-term pathogenesis of the illness. But a sudden reduction in drinking among "people already predisposed to die from cardiovascular disease (for instance, cardiac patients) could certainly induce a rapid decrease in their mortality" (Shkolnikov and Meslé 1996:133).

After the anti-alcohol campaign was terminated in 1987 because of its widespread public unpopularity, alcohol consumption increased and life expectancy decreased again—falling from 64.9 years for males in 1987 to 63.5 years in 1991. Shkolnikov and Nemtsov (1994:1) conclude that "the rapid mortality decrease in the years 1984 to 1987 can be assumed to reflect a pure effect of reduced alcohol abuse on mortality because there were no other significant changes in conditions of public health in that short period." When the Soviet state fell apart and the populace was subjected to radical social and economic changes, longevity turned lower once again. Shkolnikov and Nemtsov find that alcohol also played a major role in rising mortality between 1988 and 1992, but in 1993 overall conditions were so bad that it is difficult to isolate the effects of drinking alone. According to Shkolnikov and Meslé (1996:133), "In 1993 the public health situation worsened so much that at first it seemed unbelievable." A return to table 4.1 in chapter 4 shows that longevity decreased 2.5 years for males and 0.9 years for females between 1993 and 1994. Between 1988 and 1991, alcohol consumption increased relatively slowly, but in 1992 drinking accelerated and most likely played a key role in the 1993 drop in life expectancy.

According to Shkolnikov and Nemtsov (1994), the style of drinking common among middle-aged Russian men is derived from a general northern European pattern featuring rapid group consumption of large doses of vodka with a light snack. The participant is expected to continue to drink with his fellows even when he feels he has had enough. Drunkenness is usually the norm on these occasions and apparently little or no stigma is associated with being intoxicated. In the late nineteenth and early twentieth centuries, Russian workers and peasants typically drank large amounts of alcohol only on their days off, namely Sundays and Russian Orthodox Church holidays. Russian anthropologist Olga Semyonova Tian-Shanskaia (1993) studied peasant life in the early 1900s and found that drinking was heavy on particular occasions, especially at weddings, street parties, and fairs. Tian-Shanskaia (1993:110–1) comments that:

> The best occasion for young people to get drunk for the first time is the annual festival, which in this region takes place in connection with St. Michael's Day. On that holiday, every person in the parish is drunk. In a good year the festival lasts for a week, but even when the crops are poor,

people manage to go on a spree for three days. There is also a great deal of drinking at Shrovetide. This is a time for traveling to visit relatives, and for riding troikas. Accidents abound in the springtime [as a result of drunkenness]. Some people drown in water-filled ravines. Others are crushed under falling wagons; a drunken peasant will have a wagon tip over on him and that is the end of him. Considerably less drinking occurs on Christmas and Easter.

What is suggested by Tian-Shanskaia's study is that episodic binge drinking during holidays was normative in peasant communities during the czarist period. However, during the Soviet era alcohol use became increasingly common throughout the year, which fostered a male lifestyle characterized by consistent rather that intermittent binge drinking. According to Specter (1997a), no country consumes more hard liquor than Russia, and this shows in their health problems. "Alcohol abuse is a direct cause," states Specter (1997a:A3), "of what demographers and politicians regard as potentially the greatest threat facing Russia: its sharp and continuing drop in life expectancy." Specter suggests that trying to reduce alcohol use in Russia is an almost futile task. Stalin considered it and decided against it. Gorbachev tried it and was ridiculed as "Mr. Mineral Water." Specter (1997a:A3) observes that in most of the world Dmitri Mendeleiev is known for devising the periodic table of elements in chemistry, but in Russia, "he is at least as well-known, and far more fondly, as the Russian who first realized that 40% is the best proportion of alcohol for vodka."

Today, public health efforts in Russia are focused on teaching children about the problems of alcohol abuse, while the government is intent on regaining lost tax revenues from alcohol sales. Drinking in Russia is economically important because in 1988 alcohol taxes comprised 35% of the Soviet government's income. Today, with most sales (70%) taking place without taxation on the black market, taxes from alcohol contribute only 5% to the national budget, causing Yeltsin's government to both double taxes on vodka and attempt to control its production and sales by unofficial sources (Specter 1997a). Thus, the effects of a traditional "macho" drinking culture are exacerbated by a reduced state control over the quality of alcohol sold in the marketplace (Ryan 1995). In sum, drinking in Russia is widespread, deadly, and exceedingly resistant to change and control.

Smoking

About 67% of the Russian population reportedly smoked in 1992, which represents a sizable increase from 1985 when that figure was 53% (Tchachenko and Riazantsev 1993). Smoking among females is much lower than among males and varies by region. In industrial areas, some 78.6% of men smoked in 1986, compared to 13.7% of women; in 1992, in Moscow, 49% of men and 9.2% of women were smokers, while in Siberia, 69.4% of men and 7.9% of women smoked (Hurt 1995; Prokhorov 1993). Additional research on Moscow provides similar figures, showing that some 46% of male and 16% of female respondents smoked daily (Palosuo et al. 1995). What is suggested by these studies is that Russian men, especially middle-aged workers, add high levels of smoking to their health lifestyles.

Western tobacco companies have been successfully targeting the Russian population as a vast, relatively new market. Western brands are preferred over Russian cigarettes, which usually have filters but a very high tar content (Hurt 1995). Western cigarettes on sale in Russia are primarily produced in Third World countries; they are inexpensive and their quality is poor. Smoking's greatest contribution to the current death rate is likely through heart disease in combination with heavy drinking. Deaths from lung cancer have barely risen from 53.2 deaths per 100,000 in 1987 to 55 in 1993, thereby suggesting that the greatest effects of smoking on lung cancer are yet to come. It has been estimated that about 20% of Russia's population will eventually die from tobacco-related causes (Peto et al. 1992).

Diet and Exercise

In the early 1990s, state subsidies for meat and other food products were removed as food markets were privatized. Higher food prices resulted, and in 1992–93, the intake of protein in Russia declined by 23% (Shkolnikov and Meslé 1996). Between 1990 and 1993, the per capita annual consumption of meat and meat products, milk and dairy products, eggs, fish, sugar, vegetable oil, and vegetables and melons decreased, and that of potatoes, bread, and pasta increased (State Committee of the Russian Federation on Statistics 1994). Although in the first year (1992) of inflated food prices there was some nutritional deprivation among the elderly (Rush and Welch 1996), there is evidence that more pensioners gained than lost weight in 1992–94 (Popkin, Zohoori, and Baturin 1996). The Russian people have not experienced food shortages and have generally maintained an adequate level of nutritional well-being, but their diet has been characterized by high animal fat intake and low levels of high-quality protein intake (Beliaev 1996; Shkolnikov and Meslé 1996). The overall food situation in Russia can be summarized as follows:

> Food supply and poor nutrition were, and continue to be, chronic problems in Russia. Healthy foods are not readily available: Meats are very fatty; fruits and vegetables are limited in supply and variety; and all foods are costly (i.e., in terms of declining average incomes). Fortification of foods with vitamins and minerals, such as iodine in salt, is practiced but not mandated or widely available. Iodine deficiency disorders are estimated to affect 30 million Russians, and other nutritional deficiency problems, including iron deficiency, anemia, and rickets, are reported common. (Tulchinsky and Varavikova 1996:316)

While there has been little research comparing the eating habits of men and women, there is evidence that within families the husband eats 50% more meat than the wife and the wife eats more fruit and about the same amount of vegetables (Shapiro 1995). Overall, men consume more fat than women and it is clear "that on average women, whose mortality rates have increased less rapidly, have kept up a far healthier diet than men" (Shapiro 1995:165). Although nutrition per se does not appear to bear major responsibility for the decline in life expectancy, the eating practices of men seem to put them at greater risk for heart disease, which, in turn, contributes to their higher mortality.

As for leisure-time exercise—the form of exercise considered most beneficial to health—there is an absence of research. What little data exist suggest that such exercise is not widely practiced in Russia. For example, in a comparison of Moscow and Helsinki residents, Hannele Palosuo (1997:7) found that: "Leisure-time physical exercise was not popular in Moscow." While only 12% of the Finnish respondents exercised less frequently than at least once a month, some 43% of the Russian men and 59% of the women put themselves in this category. Better educated men in Moscow exercised the most, and the occupational group least prone to exercise—not surprisingly, given their high mortality rate—were industrial workers. Despite the importance of physical culture and sports participation for health in Russia, the overall proportion of the population that engages in such activities is low—an estimated 21% of all males and 12% of females (Field 1995; Rimachevskaya 1993).

Empirical Data

Analysis of data from the Russian Longitudinal Monitoring Survey (RLMS) provides empirical evidence in support of the lifestyle pattern just outlined. This survey, an ongoing project since 1992, has been a cooperative effort of the Carolina Population Center at the University of North Carolina at Chapel Hill, the Institute of Sociology of the Russian Academy of Sciences, the Institute of Nutrition of the Russian Academy of Medical Sciences, and Paragon Research International. This is a randomly selected, nationally representative survey of the effects of the post-communist Russian reforms on the health and economic well-being of both households and individuals. The data analyzed in table 5.4 are based on the responses of 8,402 individuals interviewed in person in 1995.

Table 5.4

Standardized Regression Coefficients (Beta) and Unstandardized Regression Coefficients (b) for Health Lifestyles, Health Status, and Life Satisfaction in Russia, 1995 (N=8,402)

	Alcohol	Smoking	Exercise	Fat Intake	Health Status	Life Satisfaction
Male	.10***	.52***	.11***	.05***	.13***	.05***
	(.52)	(.48)	(.23)	(.10)	(.20)	(.10)
Age	-.10***	-.11***	-.21***	-.09***	-.48***	-.13***
	(-.01)	(-.00)	(-.05)	(-.04)	(-.02)	(-.00)
Education	.09***	-.05***	.06***	.10***	.05***	.03***
	(.13)	(-.01)	(.03)	(.56)	(.02)	(.01)
Income	.05***	.02	.05***	.06***	.01	.11***
	(.00)	(.00)	(.00)	(.00)	(.00)	(.00)
Urban	.03**	.03**	.09***	.03**	.35	.06***
	(.15)	(.00)	(.20)	(.69)	(.00)	(.14)
Married	.08***	.01	-.12***	.03**	.47	-.18
	(.41)	(.00)	(-.26)	(.59)	(.00)	(-.00)
Employed	.15***	.08***	-.07**	.04***	.08***	-.01
	(.73)	(.07)	(-.14)	(.81)	(.12)	(-.03)
Constant	1.80	.19	.85	31.23	3.83	2.33
R^2	.10	.32	.09	.04	.31	.04

* = p < .05, ** = p < .01, *** = p < .001

The sample was 56.5% female and 43.5% male. Ages ranged from 16 to 102 years, with a mean age of 44.8 years. Some 21% of the respondents had not completed secondary school or any technical training courses, while 14.6% were university, institute, or academy graduates. The mean for completed education was between that of a secondary (high school) graduate and professional/technical trade school/factory training graduate without secondary education. The mean income for the last 30 days, computed in dollars at the exchange rate for the period, was $80.09. As for employment, some 51.3% were employed outside the home and 48.7% were housewives or unemployed. In addition, some 63.1% were married and some 74.4% lived in urban areas.

Seven independent variables were used in the analysis. *Male*, coded as males = 1 and females = 0; *age*, coded in years; *education*, coded by type of formal schooling completed; *income*, as indicated by total individual income in the last 30 days; *urban*, coded as urban = 1, rural = 0; *married*, coded as married = 1, unmarried = 0; and *employed*, coded as employed = 1, unemployed = 0. Four indices were constructed to serve as dependent variables and measures of health lifestyles. *Alcohol* measures frequency of drinking and is an ordinal scale based on responses to the question "How often have you used alcoholic beverages in the last 30 days?" Alcohol is coded do not drink = 0, drank once in the last 30 days = 1, drank 2–3 times in the last 30 days = 2, drank once a week = 3, drank 2–3 times a week = 4, drank 4–6 times a week = 5, and drank every day = 6. *Smoking* measures use of cigarettes and is coded never smoked = 0, former smoker = 1, and current smoker = 2. *Exercise* measures leisure-time (recreational) exercise and is coded no exercise = 0, light physical exercise less than 3 times a week = 1, medium intensive exercise less than 3 times a week = 2, intensive exercise at least 3 times a week = 3, and daily exercise = 4. *Fat intake* measures the average daily percentage of calories from fat consumed by the respondent and is a specially constructed data set based on dietary journals maintained by the respondents. Scores range from .44 to 77.1.

Two other dependent variables are health status and life satisfaction. *Health status* is a subjective self-ranking of one's own health and consists of a 5-point Likert scale in which the range of responses are coded very bad = 1, bad = 2, average (not good but not bad) = 3, good = 4, and very good = 5. *Life satisfaction* measures responses to the question "To what extent are you satisfied with your life in general at the present time?" Responses are coded not at all satisfied = 5, less than satisfied = 4, both yes and no = 3, rather satisfied = 2, and fully satisfied = 1. Means, standard deviations, and correlation coefficients are shown in the appendix. Data are analyzed by multiple regression.

Table 5.4 presents regression results for health lifestyles, self-assessments of health status, and perceived life satisfaction. Males are significantly more likely than females to engage in all four of the health lifestyle behaviors by drinking alcohol more frequently, being a smoker, exercising, and consuming higher amounts of fat. Whereas exercise is a positive activity, few Russians appear to do it on a regular basis. Only 21.9% of the respondents exercised at all. Results indicate that among the Russians who do exercise, there is a significantly greater proportion of men than women. Despite the more frequent drinking, smoking, and high fat intake, the males in this sample were more likely to rate their health status and life satisfaction high. It is possible that drinking and smoking with their fellows promotes a sense of well-being among these men, despite the implications for their future health status and longevity. This suggests either a lack of knowledge (or awareness) about the effects of unhealthy lifestyle practices on their bodies, or a disregard that could ultimately prove fatal.

Age has significant effect on all four health lifestyle variables, as well as on health status and life satisfaction, with younger respondents scoring higher on all measures. Given the mean age of 44.8 years, these results indicate that it is the middle-aged who are producing much of the differences. A separate examination of drinking and smoking by age-groups not shown in table 5.4, for example, indicates that drinking among Russian males begins in earnest at ages 20–24 and climbs steadily to its peak between ages 35 and 39, before decreasing slightly in the 40–44 and 45–49 age-groups. From age 50 onward, drinking declines significantly. Of course, many Russian men are dead by their mid- to late 50s. Smoking is common from ages 20 to 49 but also declines after age 50, perhaps for the same reason (those who smoke frequently are dead or dying). The greatest prevalence of smoking is found among the 30- to 34-year-olds, but this lead—in comparison to other age groups with large proportion of smokers—is slight.

The results for education show that lower-educated people are more likely to smoke. On the other hand, higher-educated people are more likely to drink, exercise, eat fat, and rate both their health and life satisfaction high. The same pattern generally exists for income, except that this variable makes no difference with respect to smoking and self-rated health status. Persons who reside in urban areas are also significantly more likely to score high on the lifestyle practices and life satisfaction, but this variable does not produce a significant effect for health status. Table 5.4 shows that marriage makes a major difference in that married people are more likely to drink and eat fatty foods, while unmarried people are more likely to exercise. Marriage is not significant with respect to smoking, self-rated health, or life satisfaction. Being married does not in itself promote healthy lifestyle practices in relation to eating and drinking, nor does it provide high life satisfaction. Thus, the quality of many Russian marriages may not be especially helpful in providing positive levels of health promotion and social support. More research is needed, however, to fully investigate the quality of Russian married life generally before making a definitive statement concerning the relationship between marital relations and health. Finally, people who are employed drink and smoke more, exercise less, have a higher fat intake, and rate their health status higher than the unemployed. Having a job does not provide greater life satisfaction.

Overall, these data do not present a positive image of Russian health lifestyles. Employed middle-aged males who live in urban areas, are married, and have higher incomes and education show the greatest consumption of alcohol and fat. The less educated in this group are more likely to smoke as well. Being married and having a job do not promote significantly greater life satisfaction—which suggests some very serious social problems in Russian society concerning marriage and work. Low social support within marriage and a lack of satisfaction at work help explain why drinking is so widespread among the men in this survey. In this context, frequent alcohol consumption with one's friends may be a preferred activity and a source of male bonding. Whatever the reason for it, drinking alcohol operates as a normative activity strongly embedded in the lifestyle of these men.

CONCLUSION: THE CAUSES
OF AN UNHEALTHY LIFESTYLE

The foregoing discussion identifies a particularly unhealthy and obviously life-shortening lifestyle among middle-aged working-class Russian males, with the world's highest per capita consumption of alcohol (usually in the form of vodka), high levels of smoking, a high-fat diet, with little fresh fruit, and little or no leisure-time exercise. Each of these are major risk factors for cardiovascular disease. Therefore, it is not coincidental that diseases of the circulatory system have become so prominent in Russia. Nor is it surprising that alcohol abuse has promoted accidents, poisonings, and injuries as the nation's second leading cause of death. As Shkolnikov (1996) explains, only two classes of causes of death have played a principal role in changes in life expectancy at birth since the 1960s—cardiovascular diseases, and external causes of death through accidents, injuries, poisonings, and violence.

Returning to Max Weber's ([1922]1978) concept of lifestyles as involving the interplay of life choices and life chances, the health lifestyle of middle-aged working-class Russian men appears to be influenced more by chance (structure) than choice (agency). Consistent with Pierre Bourdieu's (1984, 1990) theoretical approach, the unhealthy lifestyle choices of these men can be seen as reflecting a habitus. This habitus is based upon the experiences, socialization, and class conditions of the men involved, with the key variables of class, age, and gender producing the most important differences between themselves and others. The result is an enduring orientation toward an unhealthy style of living that becomes routine and, when acted on continuously, reproduces itself over time. Or, in Bourdieu's (1990:53) terms, it is a system of durable and structured structures predisposed to operate as structuring structures.

Excessive alcohol use, for example, stems from the normative demand of this particular Russian male lifestyle—that is, heavy and frequent episodic drinking is a strong tradition of peasant and working-class culture and, in this context, is not an entirely free lifestyle choice (Cockerham 1997; Palosuo 1997; Ryan 1995). While one might argue that these men drink because they want to, not because they have to, the fact remains that the norms and interpersonal dynamics of their group force them to choose to drink, if they wish to belong and freely participate in the company of their friends, which in essence amounts to not having a choice at all. This drinking tradition qualifies as a structural constraint limiting choice. Male drinking in Russia is therefore bound up in the culture, norms, values, and group dynamics of middle-aged workers. Gorbachev's short-lived anti-alcohol campaign consisted of only two measures—limiting production and raising prices. Alcohol consumption dropped not because of a choice made by drinkers (who objected to the campaign and secured its discontinuation in 1987), but because of the material constraint of alcohol shortage.

It is not as certain whether group norms are as strong and pervasive for smoking as they are for drinking. However, the well-established association between cigarette and alcohol consumption, along with reports that almost 80% of the adult males in industrial areas smoke (Hurt 1995), link smoking to the normative framework of male working-class lifestyles. Diet is another lifestyle behavior in which choice has been traditionally limited because of the lessened availability of health-promoting foods. As for leisure-time exercise, this lifestyle does not support it. These men have the option to exercise but do not utilize it (which could be construed as a choice).

If lifestyles are social constellations of style and activity whose parameters are established by a particular habitus and channel behavior down a prescribed path, then the lifestyle of the middle-aged working-class Russian male sets the people it represents on a course to poor health. Part of the responsibility for this situation lies in the patronage orientation of the former Soviet state. According to Boris Rozenfeld (1996:164), everyone was under the umbrella of the central government, which undertook the entire responsibility for their health. This situation, Rozenfeld suggests, fostered an irresponsible attitude by individuals as they delegated fully to the state the right to define and provide for their health needs. This means that participating in a healthy lifestyle was neither encouraged nor rewarded. The idea that individuals were ultimately responsible for their own health because of the limits of medicine and the importance of lifestyles for health was not popularized. Soviet society placed a low value on the individual and the individual's health (Field 1995). The needs of the collective were seen as vastly more important in building socialism than the needs of the individual. As Shkolnikov and Meslé (1996:145) put it:

> The priority of state aims and interests over personal needs and wishes taught people that their individual values were of minor importance. According to this ideology, there was no reason to pay much attention to one's future health. Many people believed that the state would help them in case of a serious health problem or any other disaster. Their resulting careless lifestyle has become especially dangerous under the new circumstances, when the general weakness of the Russian state has made its social and health efforts even more inadequate than in previous years.

The residual psychological effects of dependence on the former Soviet state and the uncertainty associated with postcommunist change may be partly responsible for undermining the motivation of individuals to pursue a healthy lifestyle in the new Russia. However, Palosuo (1997:10) found that the health-promoting activities of men in Helsinki were more affected by a sense of powerlessness and hopelessness than men in

Moscow. Overall, there is a lack of evidence blaming the downturn in life expectancy on the above-mentioned psychological causes, and the paternalism of the state seems to have had its greatest health effect on promoting false security and careless behavior (Shkolnikov and Meslé 1996). The studies discussed in this chapter lead to the conclusion that the health lifestyle of middle-aged working-class Russian males is the primary social determinant of the decline in longevity. This lifestyle, which provides the behavioral parameters for drinking, smoking, diet, and exercise, survived the transition from communism to postcommunism without major modifications. Today it operates as a deadly force shortening the lifespan of those who follow its norms.

Chapter 6

Hungary

First in the discussion of Eastern Europe is Hungary, whose health profile has been the poorest among the former socialist countries outside the former Soviet Union. Although they shared the same communist ideology, the Eastern European socialist countries were not a unified group; they had different cultures, historical traditions, social problems, and national experiences (Ostrowska 1996). These countries also differed with respect to the degree of agricultural collectivization, the extent of popular support for the state, the existence of independent social groups outside the Communist Party, the commitment to communism, and the operation of market mechanisms to supplement central planning (Wong 1995). Hungary, in particular, is different because it once was a prominent member of one of Europe's major empires—the Austro-Hungarian, or Habsburg, Empire—which lasted into the early twentieth century and stretched across a vast territory in both Eastern and Western Europe. Consequently, Hungary has closer historical ties to the West than most other former socialist countries.

As in the last chapter, I begin the discussion by examining the relationship between health and social change in Hungary and then review the health effects of policy, societal stress, and lifestyles in the search for the primary social determinant for the downturn in life expectancy.

This chapter was written with the assistance of Péter Józan, M.D., Ph.D., Head, Division of Population and Health Statistics, Hungarian Central Statistical Office, Budapest, Hungary.

HEALTH AND SOCIAL CHANGE IN HUNGARY

In order to place Hungary's current health profile into perspective, I will open with an account of the nation's social history in relation to patterns of life expectancy. Hungary had been a medieval kingdom when most of the country was conquered by the Turks in 1526. After nearly 200 years of continued warfare, Hungary was acquired in 1699 by Austria's Habsburg dynasty. As part of the Habsburg Empire, Hungary maintained its identity as a distinct kingdom and its ruling class enjoyed a relatively free hand governing within its borders. In 1867 Austria and Hungary were united as a dual monarchy, with each country having its own constitution and parliament but joined together under the rule of the Habsburg emperor, Franz Josef. The merger with Austria gave Hungary a boost in economic development and initiated a social transition in the emergence of a professional middle class, a decline in the number of peasants, and the rise of an urban industrial working class (Kolosi and Szelényi 1993). At the end of the nineteenth century, Austria-Hungary was a huge multiethnic state and a major European power, whose lands—in addition to Austria and Hungary—included the present-day nations of Croatia, Bosnia, Romania, Slovenia, and the Czech and Slovak Republics, as well as parts of Italy, Poland, and the Ukraine.

The Late Imperial Period

In 1900, Hungary's capital, Budapest, was one of the great cities of Europe. It was economically prosperous and had an active literary, artistic, and cultural life. According to American historian John Lukacs (1988:14), a native of Budapest, "Foreign visitors arriving in that unknown portion of Europe, east of Vienna, were astounded to find a modern city with first-class hotels, plate-glass windows, electric tramcars, elegant men and women, the largest Parliament building in the world about to be completed." Budapest also had a very class-conscious society. At the top of Hungary's social structure was the old feudal nobility of large landowners whose wealth was primarily based on agriculture and forestry. As Lukacs points out, the upper-class nobility married mostly among themselves, although some intermarriages with wealthy banking and industrial families had begun as capitalism was starting to transform the economy. Next in the social order was a less affluent landed gentry—a *petite noblesse*—who lacked the riches and power of the class above them, but still had their titles and were popularly regarded as socially superior to the classes below them (Lukacs 1988). One of the major changes in Hungarian society at this time was the movement of many sons and daughters of the gentry into the upper-middle class as they increasingly moved into the ranks of the professions (Kolosi and Szelényi 1993). Far wealthier, but not yet as high on the social scale as the gentry, were an affluent group of leading bankers, merchants, factory owners, and urban landlords. Below them was a growing upper and lower middle class, followed by an established working class of urban industrial workers and domestic servants. At the bottom of society was a large lower class of peasants in the countryside and unskilled urban laborers like street cleaners, garbage men, and janitors.

Table 6.1

Life Expectancy at Birth in Hungary, 1900–1997

Year	Males	Female
1900–01	36.6	38.2
1920–21	41.0	43.3
1930–31	48.7	51.8
1941	55.0	58.2
1949	59.3	63.4
1960	65.9	70.1
1966	67.5	72.2
1970	66.3	72.1
1980	65.4	72.7
1985	65.1	73.1
1986	65.3	73.2
1987	65.7	73.7
1988	66.1	74.0
1989	65.4	73.8
1990	65.1	73.7
1991	65.0	73.8
1992	64.5	73.7
1993	64.5	73.8
1994	64.8	74.2
1995	65.2	74.5
1996	66.1	74.7
1997	66.3	75.1

SOURCE: Hungarian Central Statistical Office 1997.

Life expectancy in 1900–01, as shown in table 6.1, was 36.6 years for males and 38.2 years for females. Eastern Europe has traditionally had lower life expectancy than Western Europe and this was also the case at the beginning of the twentieth century. French men, for example, lived an average of 43.4 years in 1900 and French women an average of 47 years. Americans had an even longer life expectancy in 1900 with 46.3 years for men and 48.3 years for women—about 10 years longer on average than the Hungarians.

Nevertheless, food was cheap in Hungary and even the poorest segment of the population ate better than the poor elsewhere in the Habsburg lands. Moreover, as Lukacs (1988:81) found, alcoholism in Budapest was not as excessive in 1900 as it was in many other major European cities. The reputation of being an alcoholic made a person socially unacceptable to the middle and upper classes. An interest in sports was also beginning to develop in 1900, especially in horse racing (among the upper and working classes) and ice skating (among the upper-middle class), while soccer was being introduced for the first time.

In 1914, Austria-Hungary declared war on Serbia after the assassination of the Habsburg archduke Francis Ferdinand in Bosnia by a member of a Serbian revolutionary society. The activation of a series of military alliances across Europe in response to this action led to World War I and the end of the Austro-Hungarian, German, and Russian Empires. In describing Budapest toward the end of the war, Lukacs (1988:210) writes: "One gets the impression that sometime in late 1917 those shafts of sunshine that illuminated, if only temporarily, the streets and the squares and even the spirit of the city during the first years of the war had disappeared; that the climate of this summery city had given way to a darkening, rain-laden and heavy; that the clocks had moved from an early afternoon to a late hour." Austria-Hungary was losing the war, and the end came in October 1918. In the subsequent peace treaty, Hungary lost two-thirds of its historic territory and half of its population—including the loss of the entire province of Transylvania to Romania. Other territory was ceded to Austria, the Ukraine, the former Czechoslovakia, the former Soviet Union, and the former Yugoslavia. According to Hungarian sociologists Tamás Kolosi and Ivan Szelényi (1993:143):

> The loss of the First World War and the breakup of the Austro-Hungarian monarchy was a deep shock for the Hungarian economy and society. The dynamic capitalist development Hungary had experienced in the past was fueled by the favorable strategic position it had gained in the region after

the agreement with Austria in 1867. For decades, Hungary had the privilege of being the "junior partner" of Austria's imperialism. After having lost this privileged position, Hungary experienced a crumbling of its economy, a flood of refugees, and massive unemployment which badly affected not only the working class, but also the professional class.

The Period between 1918 and 1945

Hungary began 1918 as a republic, but a communist takeover resulted in a brief (132 days) Hungarian Soviet Republic that, in turn, was overthrown by counterrevolutionaries who tried but failed to restore the Habsburg monarchy. In 1920, Hungary emerged as a democratic monarchy with a perennially vacant throne; however, the government was controlled by Miklós Horthy, a former rear admiral of the Austro-Hungarian navy. Hungary had a constitution, parliament, elections, and multiple political parties, but in reality it was a dictatorship. Life began returning to normal, however, and a measure of financial stability and economic development reappeared. As seen in table 6.1, between 1920–21 and 1941 life expectancy for males increased from 41 years to 55 years and for females from 43.1 years to 58.2 years. This indicates an increasingly positive health situation in Hungary at that time.

Hungary's traditional social structure remained generally intact during the years before World War II. Land reform had little success. The old landed nobility remained powerful, and by 1930 a third of the cultivated land was still owned by only a few hundred families. According to Hungarian sociologist Ferenc Erdei (1988), capitalism had penetrated the country but had not transformed society; rather, the traditional feudal social structure had survived. When land was given to peasants, the new owners often lacked the capital and knowledge for private farming, and agricultural production did not rise appreciably. Hungarian agriculture was, in fact, badly hurt by the worldwide economic depression that began in 1929, but the economy in general improved after 1933. However, Hungary's situation was to worsen when the country became a German ally in World War II and joined in the 1941 invasion of the Soviet Union. With the war effort going poorly by 1944 and the Soviet Army advancing to the border, the Hungarian government sought to change sides. But the Germans occupied Budapest until driven out by the Russians in February 1945, the city was heavily destroyed. As Lukacs (1988:220) describes it, the bridges and many of the famous buildings were in ruins; only 26 of every hundred buildings remained relatively intact; nearly all of the windows in Budapest were broken, and electricity, gas, and telephones were nonexistent.

The Communist Period

After a temporary period of transitory and restricted democracy, Hungary became a socialist state under the control of its Communist Party in 1948. The remnants of the old nobility lost their land and power as the large feudal estates were dismantled (Kolosi and Szelényi 1993). Many surviving members of the upper and middle classes left the country; others were arrested and imprisoned, or deported as enemies of the state. The communist regime, dominated by the Soviet Union, was highly unpopular and its legitimacy was increasingly questioned. On 23 October 1956, armed revolt broke out in the streets of Budapest. The Soviet forces were driven out of the city for a few days, but a counterattack on 3–4 November quelled the uprising after heavy fighting. A new communist government was installed. Over 180,000 Hungarians fled the country across the Austrian border. Yet the new regime under János Kádár did not generally (there were some exceptions) reimpose police state repression. Instead, a limited degree of individual and cultural freedom was allowed within the constraints of a communist dictatorship. As Kolosi and Szelényi (1993:146) point out: "A neo-Stalinist rule came to power, but only for a few years, and as early as in the beginning of the 1960s the new Hungarian ruling elite was ready to compromise with different social forces within the society."

Hungary's class structure was altered to reflect the country's socialist orientation. The Communist Party (the Hungarian Socialist Workers Party), as in the other former socialist countries, adopted policies to "destratify" society for political, ideological, and economic purposes (Wong 1995). The changes favored the working class and the peasants, while eliminating the formerly privileged social position of the nobility and the gentry. Skilled industrial workers and miners were among the best-paid people in society and the majority of managers in state-owned enterprises were recruited from their ranks. As in the other communist states, the top of the social hierarchy was occupied by the party elite, and the lower strata were the working class and peasantry. In between the ruling elite and the lower strata was a rising professional middle class of technical specialists in a variety of fields.

As American sociologist Raymond Wong (1995) explains, Hungary was less ideological and more pragmatic in its approach to building socialism than its more conservative neighbors like Czechoslovakia and East Germany. Some self-employment, both full- and part-time, was allowed and in time became a "second economy," generating about one-third of the national income in the 1980s (Stokes 1993). Moreover, members of the intelligentsia—notably economists and other technically trained people—were included in the central planning processes for the state enterprises. Nonparty members were able to achieve public positions, and admission to universities was not restricted to the children of communist workers and peasants as they were often elsewhere. Peasants on the collective farms were allocated small household plots to grow vegetables to sell for personal profit in town markets. This means that many features of an open society were developed in Hungary prior to the collapse of communism, which made the transition to postcommunism easier. According to American historian Gale Stokes (1993:86):

> Looking back, it seems clear that the Hungarian reforms set the stage for relatively good economic development after 1989. But at the time, what most Hungarians noticed was a declining standard of living. . . . In Hungary price changes took place periodically and usually with lengthy preliminary preparations. This more sensible policy prevented sudden outbursts of rage but not a steady deterioration of morale, since . . . [spending power was declining]. A significant portion of the population was prosperous in the private sector, but a majority was feeling pinched by the falling value of real wages. Rising prices also reduced the value of social benefits, and those on pensions particularly suffered.

The Kádár regime had been unable to cope with the nation's economic difficulties and mounting financial debt. Allowing limited and small-scale private enterprise was not enough to offset declining productivity in the state sector. Hungary needed markets in Western Europe; to obtain these markets they needed to shift from a planned to a market economy, but the party leadership could not reform the system entirely because of ideological and bureaucratic barriers (Skidelsky 1995). By 1988, Kádár had been deposed as younger, more reform-oriented communists came to power. This happened in the face of widespread disenchantment with communism as opposition groups like the Hungarian Democratic Forum, Alliance of Free Democrats, and Alliance of Young Democrats were openly critical of the government.

With Mikhail Gorbachev actively encouraging reform in the Soviet Union and guaranteeing that Eastern Europe was free to pursue its own destiny, Hungary was the first former socialist country to renounce one-party rule and authorize multiparty elections. This decision set the stage for a public rejection of communism through the ballot box, and in 1989 Hungary left the Soviet orbit to become a multiparty parliamentary democracy with a free-market economy. Although events in some other Eastern European countries would be more dramatic in the overthrow of communism, Hungarian political reforms, along with reforms in Poland, set the revolutionary agenda that ended one-party rule in Eastern Europe (Glenny 1993; Stokes 1993). "In Hungary," states Stokes (1993:78), "János Kádár's politics of reconciliation permitted the growth of a significant autonomous sector in the Hungarian economy, the re-emergence of reformers in the party itself, and the elaboration of a set of popular issues that mobilized urban segments of the society in favor of change."

But while Hungarians were struggling with economic and political change, their health situation worsened. Between 1948 and 1989 Hungary operated a Soviet-style health care delivery system characterized by central planning and control, subsidized by the state, and providing free health care to the general population under the Uniform State Health Service Act of 1950. This act officially eliminated independent health insurance funds and made free health care a right of all citizens. Private medical practice was not forbidden but in reality was very limited. As in the Soviet Union, the health system was financed out of the central government's budget. Thus, the state funded the operation of health facilities, paid providers a salary, and set policy.

However, as a nonproductive sector of the economy, the health care delivery system began receiving a lower priority and budget in the late 1960s as economic difficulties emerged (Makara 1994). In 1971, for example, Hungary spent only 3.2% of its GDP on health care; by 1989 health spending had increased to 4.6% of the GDP, but this amount was still below what was needed to cope with the nation's health problems (Marrée and Groenewegen 1997). In order to obtain more personalized health services, the Hungarians, like people in the other socialist countries, resorted to the direct payment of gratuities and gifts to health care providers (Csaszi 1990). While this practice may have helped some patients to receive better care, Peter Makara (1994) claims that it contributed to the interests of some members of the medical profession to focus more on the treatment of diseases than their prevention since they could make more money this way.

Officially, the Hungarian health care system, like the Soviet one, was oriented toward prevention, especially secondary prevention provided by medical doctors as opposed to primary prevention in the form of promoting healthier lifestyles. As Makara (1994:1298) explains: "The existing Soviet type network was not prepared to take the lead in managing the primary prevention of chronic non-communicable diseases whose incidence was growing, nor adopt the ideas of health promotion." In the early period of communist rule, the Soviet-style approach worked—just as it did in the former Soviet Union. As shown in table 6.1, life expectancy for Hungarian men increased from 59.3 years in 1949 to 67.5 years in 1966—the highest male longevity ever recorded in that country. Life expectancy for Hungarian women improved from 63.4 years to 72.2 years over the same period. Yet, a downturn in male longevity set in after 1966, and by 1989 life expectancy had fallen to 65.4 years. For women, however, life expectancy climbed to 74 years in 1988, only to drop back slightly to 73.8 years in 1989.

The Postcommunist Period

Hungary's effort to end communism began with negotiations between the communist leaders and opposition groups demanding free, multiparty elections. Gorbachev's speech at the United Nations on 7 December 1988 was a clear indication that he rejected the use of the Soviet Union's military power as an instrument of foreign policy and supported freedom of choice as a basis for social development in both capitalist and socialist systems (Gorbachev 1996). "Given all these green lights," states Stokes (1993:99), "the surprising thing is not that Hungary continued on its path toward pluralization but that with the exception of Poland it was the only East European country to do so." The Hungarian Communist Party, dominated by reform communists and trying to stay in power by responding to the public mood, agreed in a series of meetings with opposition groups in 1989 to not only accept but sponsor a constitutional multiparty system. They believed they had enough popular support to win an open election, although it was a high-stakes gamble which they eventually lost.

Ultimately, the principal political issue centered on whether the president should be elected by the direct vote of the people or by parliament. The communists favored the former since public opinion polls showed a majority of the population would support them; most opposition groups wanted a president elected by parliament who would be easier to vote out of office if he or she became a threat to democracy. The question was put to the nation in a referendum on 26 November 1989. The election was very close, and it was a disaster for the government as the opposition won by only some 6,100 votes: The president was to be elected by parliament. Instead of being returned to office on a wave of appreciation for bringing about change, the communists had to wait for the parliamentary elections in early 1990 along with the other political parties to see if they would remain in power (Stokes 1993:138). The longer the wait, the more people realized they wanted a major change from the past, and the Communist Party (now called the Hungarian Socialist Party) won only 8.5% of the seats in the new parliament. Hungary was now a liberal democracy and one that would be invited to join the North Atlantic Treaty Organization (NATO) in 1997 and to discuss membership in the European Union in 1998.

Hungary did not engage in "shock therapy" to immediately reform its economy, but took a more gradual approach. Some free-market activities already existed and foreign investments were obtained more readily than in most other former socialist countries (Holmes 1997; Skidelsky 1995). By 1994, about 55% of Hungary's economy had been privatized and this process continues today. Initially, in the early 1990s, Hungary experienced high monetary inflation and a decline in the GDP, but by the mid-1990s (1994–96) inflation was coming down and the GDP was showing a 2 to 3% annual growth, thereby signaling that perhaps the worst was over for the economy.

It is not clear whether or not the worst is over for life expectancy. As seen in table 6.1, male longevity in Hungary continued its decline from 65.4 years in 1989 to 64.5 years in both 1992 and 1993; by 1997, however, it had improved to 66.3 years. Female longevity floated between 73.7 and 73.8 years between 1990 and 1993, but like for males, turned upward in 1994, reaching 75.1 years in 1997. Life expectancy for Hungarian females in 1997 is the highest ever recorded in Hungary. But, again, the question has to be asked whether the increases in life expectancy are due to rising longevity or to the fact that the most unhealthy people have already died? Given current longevity trends and the improved social and economic conditions in the country, it appears that Hungarians are moving toward an end in the long-term decline in male life expectancy. While it is too early to prove the accuracy of this statement, it is highly probable that the increases in life expectancy reflect rising longevity.

HUNGARIAN MORTALITY

A review of the major causes of death in Hungary suggests that the nation's health problems are far from over. As shown in table 6.2, mortality from all causes, except tuberculosis, was much higher in 1994 than in either 1947 or 1955. Heart disease, lung cancer, and cirrhosis of the liver all show an unbroken upward trend that has impacted strongly on overall male life expectancy since 1966. According to Hungarian epidemiologist Péter Józan (1996b:13):

> The male probability of dying between the ages 35-65 is at a level characteristic of the 1920s and 30s. For some groups of middle-aged men in this country, mortality is now among the worst in the world. The extremely high mortality and consequent low life expectancy are signs that, in this respect, Hungary has slipped into the Third World.

Table 6.2

Mortality Rates for Selected Major Causes of Death per 100,00 Males, Hungary, 1947–1994

Causes of Death	1947	1955	1964	1975	1980	1990	1994
Tuberculosis	141.4	50.7	43.5	20.9	18.3	10.8	10.3
Cancer of trachea, bronchus, and lung	17.4	29.1	46.8	62.2	84.1	113.6	122.1
Ischemic heart disease	—	119.2	153.2	314.0	318.0	332.6	345.8
Stroke	124.5	170.5	180.3	193.1	250.7	211.1	196.5
Liver disease and cirrhosis	8.7	10.2	13.0	26.5	42.0	76.8	129.9
Traffic accidents	—	11.7	14.7	28.2	25.6	38.7	25.6
Suicide	44.3	34.5	44.9	58.7	67.7	61.4	56.1

SOURCE: Hungarian Central Statistical Office 1996.

Table 6.3 shows that Hungarian females have essentially the same mortality pattern as the males, but much lower death rates. For females, heart disease mortality rose from 88.5 deaths per 100,000 in 1955 to 181.5 in 1994, but this increase is well below that of men for whom the rate increased from 119 per 100,000 to 345.8 during the same period. For females stroke is also the second leading killer (135.5 deaths per 100,000), but, like for males, its threat is decreasing. Also, like for males, mortality from lung cancer and cirrhosis of the liver is rising, while deaths from tuberculosis, traffic accidents, and suicide are decreasing. Mortality from breast cancer, however, rose from 12 deaths per 100,000 in 1947 to 35.4 in 1994.

Table 6.3

Mortality Rates for Selected Major Causes of Death per 100,00 Females, Hungary, 1947–1994

Causes of Death	1947	1955	1964	1975	1980	1990	1994
Tuberculosis	95.0	25.1	14.6	6.3	5.4	2.6	2.1
Cancer of trachea, bronchus, and lung	5.2	7.5	11.0	11.9	15.1	22.6	25.3
Breast cancer	12.0	17.2	19.4	27.6	29.0	32.3	35.4
Ischemic heart disease	—	88.5	86.5	191.7	162.0	171.3	181.5
Stroke	107.3	165.4	164.0	158.2	194.1	153.1	135.5
Liver disease and cirrhosis	3.7	5.8	6.1	10.7	15.6	29.3	40.5
Traffic accidents	—	2.3	3.3	7.2	7.0	11.5	7.4
Suicide	16.1	14.6	17.5	20.4	24.6	18.8	14.6

SOURCE: Hungarian Central Statistical Office 1996.

A look at both tables 6.2 and 6.3 shows that mortality from heart disease literally soared for both men and women between 1964 and 1975. Józan (1989) points out that about half of this extraordinarily high increase is probably artificial because of changes in diagnosing and coding procedures. While heart disease was important, stroke, lung cancer, suicide, and cirrhosis of the liver played important roles in driving mortality rates up as well. But while heart disease may not have accelerated as rapidly as tables 6.2 and 6.3 indicate, it is clear that this ailment is the nation's leading killer for both men and women and has indeed increased over the years. As Józan (1996b) observes, in 1994, 1 out of every 5 males who died in Hungary died of heart disease.

Like in the other former socialist countries the downturn in longevity in Hungary is concentrated among middle-aged working-class males (Carlson 1989; Orosz 1990). Overall, people at the bottom of the social hierarchy have a higher mortality than people at the top, with the gypsy population presumably having a much higher mortality than the non-gypsies (Józan 1996b). Death rates are also higher, particularly for males, in small towns and villages rather than in cities. Józan reports that the highest mortality rates are found in northeastern Hungary in the counties of Szabolcs-Szatmár-Bereg and Borsod-Abúj-Zemplén. These counties border the Ukraine and Slovakia, respectively. "In Szabolcs-Szatmár-Bereg county," states Józan (1996b:16), "the probability that a 35-year-old man will reach his 65th birthday is more than 50% lower than the national average at the turn of the century." It is therefore not surprising that Hungary's population is declining. In 1996, Hungary had a population of 10.2 million people. This was 33,000 fewer people than in 1995, which is only the most recent year of a long-term population decline after 1980 when the nation had 10.7 million inhabitants. Replacing the number of people in the population is not an easy task because the mortality rate is much higher than the birth rate. In 1995, for example, there were 15.8 deaths versus 11 births per 1,000 population. Consequently, the poor health of the population is having profound effects upon Hungary. As Józan (1996b:15) explains:

> The crisis of health is not a Hungarian peculiarity. Every former socialist country east of the Elbe is having to face a similar crisis. But it is remarkable that—with the exception of some states of the former Soviet Union and certain regions of the Russian Federation—the health crisis is nowhere more serious than here in Hungary.

THE SOCIAL DETERMINANTS OF LIFE EXPECTANCY

As in Russia and elsewhere in Eastern Europe, the downturn in life expectancy in Hungary is grounded in social rather than biomedical causes. Neither infectious disease, genetic maladaptation, environmental pollution, nor inferior health care appear to be the major sources of the nation's health problems. It is true that Hungary has serious pollution problems, including poor air quality from automobile emissions in Budapest and toxic discharges into the air and ground waters in industrial areas. But environmental pollution is not primarily responsible for the continuing increase in middle-age male mortality (Hertzman 1995). And, while estimates of the number of avoidable deaths due to poor responses from the health care delivery system range from 12 to 18% of deaths annually (Forster and Józan 1990; Józan 1996b), Hungary's health services are not the cause of the heart disease, stroke, lung cancer, and liver cirrhosis that are the ultimate origin of the high death rates. Thus, in the search for the primary determinant of the increased mortality I return to policy, societal stress, and health lifestyles.

Policy

As stated previously, Hungary's health care delivery system undoubtedly contributed to the decline in life expectancy because of its inadequacy in coping with the rise of chronic diseases in the population at large, and especially with respect to containing the rise of heart disease, lung cancer, and alcohol-related deaths among men. Hungarian sociologist Eva Orosz (1990) suggests that the deterioration of the health care system needs to be viewed from a systemic perspective. The inefficient, nonmarket, state-run economy drained resources that could have been used elsewhere, such as for improving health care. State ownership of the health care delivery system also led to a rigid institutional structure that was unable to adjust to new conditions, like the rise in heart disease. "These two factors," states Orosz (1990:856), "the lack of resources and the rigid institutional structures, constitute the main reasons for the malfunctioning of the health-care system." Interwoven in this situation were various dysfunctional aspects of the political and economic features of socialism, such as rigid central planning, devaluation of the individual in favor of the collective, fiscal priority to the military and to heavy industry, and disregard for the natural environment.

Hungary's health policy, as in the other socialist states, was oriented toward providing a basic level of free care to the population in general and a higher (but unpublicized) level of services to the ruling elite. But health care was not a policy priority; its overall goals were unclear, and its general quality was considerably poorer than that available in the West (Csaszi 1990; Józan 1996b; Makara 1994; Orosz, 1990, 1996). Inferior health services generated by state policy most likely contributed to the premature deaths of some individuals. Yet, again, it was not medical care that killed so many people, especially middle-aged working-class males. Over 80% of the deaths cannot be attributed to avoidable mortality associated with health practitioners and facilities (Józan 1996b). Still, the proportion of avoidable deaths is too high for a developed society and the generally poor reputation of the health services, along with the reality of the population's extensive health problems, has led to reforms in the postcommunist era. The Local Governments Act of 1990 shifted the ownership of hospitals from the central government to local governments in order to secure better response to local needs. Most of the hospital operating costs still come from the central government, however. Polyclinics are administered by hospitals and patients can use them only on a referral from a family doctor (Roemer 1994). There is also a Health Insurance Fund operated by the Ministry of Health, which is supported by contributions from employers (18% of wages) and employees (4% of wages) and funds health services for workers. Other money to support medical treatment comes from the government's central budget and from out-of-pocket costs to patients. Health expenditures by the government have increased, reaching a high of 7.3% of the GDP in 1994. In 1996, the most recent year for which data are available, 6.7% of the GDP was spent on health. These figures do not include gratuities from patients which still exist and most likely push health spending up another 1% of the GDP. Physicians are still paid a salary by the government which in 1994 was between $125 and $185 per month (the minimum wage at that time was $110 per month). According to Dutch researchers Jörgen Marrée and Peter Groenewegen (1997:88–89):

> To boost their income, [Hungarian] physicians still ask their patients for gratitude money in exchange for better treatment. Because health care personnel are salaried and receive a guaranteed income, they have no incentive to work more efficiently. The gratitude money stimulates physicians to treat as many patients as possible, especially rich patients whom the medical staff can persuade to offer high under-the-table payments.

Consequently, the income of physicians remains embedded in the former socialist system as doctors are paid a relatively small salary and look to patients to provide them with extra money for better service. As Orosz (1996) points out, Hungary's effort to finance its health care system remains somewhat disorganized and temporary. The Health Insurance Fund has been operating at a deficit, since income from employers and employees have not kept up with expenses. Whereas there has been a cap on payments to providers under a system of DRGs (Diagnostic Related Groups) which stipulates how much the government will pay for specific services, costs for pharmaceuticals, sick pay, and pensions for disabilities have been rising. Very few doctors have privatized their practice because private medical care is not yet covered by the state's health insurance program. At present, the exact form of Hungary's health care system and its future policy has not been established.

Societal Stress

Assessing the effects of macro-level stress on the health of the Hungarian population is difficult because of a lack of data. It is certain that Hungarians have been subjected to stressful circumstances by Stalinist-type terror tactics, including arrests and executions, in the 1950s and in the aftermath of the 1956 rebellion, by deteriorating social and economic conditions under communism, and by the shock of postcommunism. It can be argued that Kádár's regime moved away from intense police-state repression and initiated reforms in return for the population's tacit approval of Kádár's government. Thus, life in Hungary may not have been subject to as much direct stress from the government as it was in other former socialist countries. Nevertheless, Makara (1994) suggests that socialism was generally stressful for Eastern Europe. He points out, though without supportive data, that extreme tension was generated in society by depressed living standards, limits on the aspirations of individuals, high workloads and low long-term rewards, and a lack of community and family social support. Yet Makara also adds that traditional risk factors like poor nutrition, lack of leisure-time exercise, smoking, and alcohol consumption cannot be overlooked. So does societal stress affect the rising mortality in some direct fashion, or does it promote premature death largely through its responsibility for unhealthy lifestyles? As stated in earlier chapters, since there is a lack of evidence that stress per se is killing people, its effects on the health of the population seem to be largely indirect, that is, through promoting too much drinking, smoking, and other unhealthy lifestyle activities.

Health Lifestyles

Once again, the principal cause of the downturn in longevity appears to be the unhealthy lifestyle of the population. Józan (1996b), for example, finds that alcoholism and smoking are the two most important risk factors in promoting increased mortality in Hungary. He estimates between 1980 and 1994, about 27% all deaths in the country were caused by excessive drinking and smoking. Two-thirds of all deaths among the 35-

to 69-year-olds in the early 1990s were attributed to smoking and alcohol consumption alone. There is evidence from several sources that during the 1970s and 1980s alcohol consumption in Hungary steadily increased and higher mortality from liver disease and cirrhosis was one of the results of this increase (Varvasovsky, Bain, and McKee 1996). As for smoking, data show that cigarette sales in Hungary and Poland were the highest in Eastern Europe from 1960 to the 1980s when Polish sales declined but Hungarian sales remained at a high plateau. And, not surprisingly, between 1985 and 1989, lung cancer for adults of both sexes between the ages of 20 and 44 was higher in Hungary than in Austria or in the rest of Eastern Europe (Kubik et al. 1995). Some 88% of the lung cancer for these men and 65% for the women were attributed to smoking. Other research investigating lung cancer in the early 1990s shows that the highest rates in Europe were among Hungarian males (Levi et al. 1995).

Another major contributor to the high mortality in Hungary is diet. Józan (1996b) observes that Hungarians consume a high level of foods containing harmful ingredients and excessive amounts of calories. A nationwide study of nutrition in 1992–94 showed that approximately 38% of the diet contained fat, primarily of animal origin with high levels of cholesterol (Biro, Antal, and Zajkas 1996), thereby suggesting that diet is a major factor in the high mortality from cardiovascular diseases (Biro 1996; Sekula, Babinska, and Petrova 1997). Other data from a cardiovascular screening program in a rural community of 2,400 inhabitants in the county of Bekes, Hungary, found a high incidence of obesity related primarily to the excessive intake of saturated animal fats (Mark, Kondacs, and Hanyecz 1997). In this village, most households cooked exclusively with animal fat, and meats with high fat content, like bacon and sausages, were popular. Again, it was concluded that nutritional factors play a major role in Hungary's high incidence of heart disease.

Some of the best evidence detailing the role of health lifestyles in Eastern Europe's mortality problems is found in Hungary's 1994 Health Behavior Survey. This survey, conducted by the Hungarian Central Statistical Office (1996), used a nationwide random sample of 5,476 households. In each household, the person with the nearest birthday, between 15 and 69 years of age, was interviewed. The findings showed that 35% of the sample were current smokers, which was about the same as in a previous 1986 survey. Since 1986, smoking had decreased among men (from 49% to 43.7%), but increased somewhat among women (from 22.4% to 26.6%). Smoking was less common among younger than older men, but for women the opposite applied. Persons with lower socioeconomic status smoked the most. Some 72% of the respondents drank alcohol regularly (84% of the men and 60% of the women) and 11.6% (primarily males) were characterized as "excessive drinkers." These data were used to estimate the proportion of alcoholics nationwide and it was projected that between the ages of 20 and 64 almost every fourth man and 2% of the women were alcoholics. Alcoholism among men was greatest in the 40–49-year-old age-group. And, unlike the Russians, who prefer vodka, beer was the most frequently consumed beverage among Hungarian men and wine was the leading choice of women.

The survey also confirmed a diet heavy in saturated fat, with pork the most popular meat and bacon one of the most common foods, especially in rural areas. Some 47.2% of the sample stated that they did not care what, how, or when they eat. Less than 10% of the men and only 12.5% of the women said they ate fresh vegetables every day in the winter. The consumption of fresh fruit almost every day in the winter was somewhat higher, with 29.4% of the men and 34.5% of the women having this positive dietary habit. As for regular physical exercise, only 21.4% of the men and 13.5% of the women had participated in this activity in the year prior to the interview. And of those who did exercise regularly, some 90% exercised only once a week. Persons with higher socioeconomic status were significantly more likely to exercise than anyone else, especially manual workers. The survey concluded that physical exercise was mainly an activity among people of school age. Furthermore, over half of all visits to physicians were made by just 10% of the respondents.

Interestingly, some 88.7% of the people surveyed were satisfied with their health lifestyle and there was no significant difference between the sexes in this regard. Józan (1996b) comments that this is surprising, given the overall state of the nation's health. "These figures," states Józan (1996b:20), "are symptomatic of ignorance among many people of what is implied by a healthy way of life." Overall, it would appear from this survey that the health lifestyle most prevalent among Hungarians is indeed the primary social determinant of the nation's rise in mortality. Smoking, alcoholism, and inadequate nutrition are blamed in the 1994 survey as the risk factors most responsible for the deterioration of health in the adult male population.

Conclusion

Midway through the communist era and into the initial postcommunist period the health of the Hungarian people has declined. Again, as in the former socialist countries generally, it is the life expectancy of middle-aged, working-class males that has been most affected. Although the results are the same, the health lifestyle components contributing the most to premature death in Hungary are somewhat different from those in the Russian experience. In Russia, the most deadly lifestyle trait is the excessive consumption of alcohol; in Hungary, the high rate of alcoholism is undoubtedly significant, but smoking is also an especially important factor in early death. Hungarians smoke more cigarettes per capita than elsewhere in Europe. In both countries, high-fat diets and low vegetable consumption in the winter, along with a general lack of leisure-time exercise, join with alcohol use and smoking to form the basis of unhealthy lifestyle practices.

It is clear that social, rather than biomedical, factors are the principal determinants of the downturn in life expectancy, with unhealthy lifestyles leading the way. These lifestyles are embedded in the social structural conditions of Hungarian life. Socialism failed to produce a healthy quality of life and to promote individual responsibility for one's own health. Too much drinking and smoking and practically no exercise became the norm among middle-aged working-class males. This, in combination with a relatively poor diet about which most people had little or no choice, evolved into a collective pattern of behavior. Although individuals have the choice of rejecting or modifying their own health lifestyle, most of them— through their habitus—tend to behave in ways that are consistent with their own routine practices and society's prevalent modes of acting.

Chapter 7

Poland

Poland never accepted communism easily but nonetheless experienced its ill effects on health. As elsewhere in the former socialist countries, mortality began rising for Polish males in the mid-1960s and was concentrated among middle-aged members of the working class. The end of communist domination came in 1989. Yet democracy did not bring an immediate halt to the downturn in life expectancy; rather, health conditions in Poland continued to deteriorate until recently. Whereas Poland's general health pattern is similar to that in the other Soviet-bloc countries, there are some important differences in the Polish experience with communism.

Three of these differences are very fundamental: Poland's religion, its Western orientation, and its free peasantry. Poland remained staunchly Roman Catholic despite communist rule. About 96% of the population today is Catholic, making the nation one of the most Catholic countries in the world, which is underscored by the fact that the current Pope, John Paul II, is Polish. The news that Poland's Cardinal Karol Wojtyla had been selected in 1978 as the first non-Italian pope in 455 years "burst like a joyous bombshell" among the Polish people and was a source of "pride and stature" for the population (Stokes 1993:33). Catholicism, therefore, served as an important presence in the daily life of the Polish people and functioned as a major counterweight to the atheistic influences of communism. According to Norman Davies (1984:11–12):

This chapter was written with the assistance of Antonina Ostrowska, Ph.D., Deputy Director, Institute of Philosophy and Sociology, Polish Academy of Sciences, Warsaw, Poland.

The position of the Roman Catholic Church in Poland after the Second World War was stronger than at any previous period of its thousand-year mission. Its strength can be explained in part by the suffering of the war years, which turned people's minds to the solace of religion: in part by the law of human cussedness, which increased people's loyalties to the Church just because their government forbade it; but largely by the ethnic and cultural remodeling of Polish society during and after the War. In 1773, . . . Polish Catholics formed barely 50% of the total population; in 1921, in the frontiers of the interwar republic, they formed 66%; in 1946, in consequence of the murder of Polish Jews by the Nazis and the expulsion of the Germans and Ukrainians, they formed no less then 96%. For the first time in history, Poland was a truly Catholic country: and it was this supercharged Catholic society which was given an atheist communist government. What a recipe!

Poland's loyalty to the Catholic Church also connected the country spiritually and culturally to the West, not the East. Identification with the traditions and culture of Latin Christianity fostered a Western outlook and sympathies well beyond any that competing influences from the East could form. Moreover, to the east lay Russia and, as Davies explains, Poland's age-old contact with the Russians had brought centuries of mistrust and bitterness. "For the Pole," states Davies (1984:345), "few things from Russia have any value—neither its shoddy manufactures, nor its ideology, nor even its superb dance, art or sport." For the Russians, in turn, nothing but trouble came out of Poland. The two countries have obviously had an uneasy relationship historically, which includes the communist period. Furthermore, Poland's major trade routes traditionally led to Western markets and back, not to Eastern ones. Although there was some commerce with Russia, Polish traders usually headed west overland to Germany or through the Baltic Sea to the Netherlands and France. As Davies (1984:343) concludes, Poland may lie geographically in the East, but in every other sense its strongest links have been with the West.

The third major difference between Poland and the rest of the former socialist countries is its free peasantry. Poland's farms were generally not collectivized except in the former German territories east of the river Oder where the large estates of the previous landowners could be easily converted to collective, state-owned farms. Under communism, over 70% of Poland's farmland—essentially small plots owned by peasants—remained in private hands. The government lacked the will and the appetite for the large-scale oppression that had occurred under Stalin in the late 1920s and the 1930s in the Ukraine, that stripped the peasants of their land and moved them onto collective farms. Still, the state controlled the prices of farm produce and the availability of agricultural machinery and fertilizers. It also made massive investments in state farming in an effort to force the less modern and relatively backward peasant farms out of business. Yet, as Davies notes, this policy turned out to be a catastrophe since the productivity of the state farms was low and the private farmers were undermined by the government. Consequently, Poland was to suffer serious food shortages. Private farming, however, survived.

Clearly, in Poland, Soviet-style communism clashed with a strong national Catholicism, traditional identification with the West, and a peasantry that generally maintained private ownership of its land. Next, I discuss Poland's historical experience in relation to health and examine the role of policy, societal stress, and health lifestyles in the country's current health situation.

HEALTH AND SOCIAL CHANGE IN POLAND

One hundred years ago, Poland did not exist as an independent nation. A series of ineffectual kings, a nobility corrupted by bribes from foreign powers, wars between other European states on Polish soil, and a troubled economy left Poland in a weakened condition. With Prussia and the Austrian and Russian Empires as its powerful neighbors, Poland needed a strong central government to defend its interests. However, this was not the case. Polish kings were elected by the nobility and their power was curtailed by the principle of *Librium Veto*, giving any member of parliament the right to veto any resolution. Behind this principle lay the honorable conviction that laws must have the consent of all those encumbered with the duty to enforce them; while there was a sense of commitment to any consensus eventually reached, Poland's parliamentary process was characterized by long debates, frequent delays, and an inability to resolve controversial issues (Davies 1984).

The potential of a stronger Poland, which occasionally surfaced when reforms were instigated or rebellions broke out, caused the country to be occupied and divided between Russia, Prussia, and Austria in three partitions occurring in 1772, 1793, and 1795. Only a small kingdom (with the Russian czar as king) remained after the third partition, but—following revolts in 1831 and 1863—this final area of Poland was converted into a Russian province and Poland disappeared from the map of

Europe. Prior to the partitions, the seat of power in Poland was occupied by only certain members of the nobility, namely by a wealthy oligarchy of magnates, as opposed to the lesser nobility who had noble titles but lacked the considerable power and riches of the magnates. The lesser nobles consisted of two groups: a less affluent landed gentry, and a landless and relatively impoverished segment of nobles. Although the magnates held the dominant role, all nobles were legally equal to each other and this right was jealously guarded. Comprising some 8 to 12% of the population, instead of the usual 1 to 2%, Poland had the highest percentage of nobles of any European country. Subordinate to the landowning nobles were the peasants, who constituted about 75% of the population. The clergy, city-dwellers, and Jews made up the other legal divisions in Polish society and were outside the direct control of the nobility, but these three mid-range social strata were too small to pose a threat to the existing social order.

Nevertheless, this feudal social structure began to change in the late nineteenth century under foreign domination. Many nobles found themselves unable to support their families from agriculture. The peasants, in turn, became more self-reliant as the power of the nobility, especially in the Prussian- and Russian-controlled areas, declined. The Prussians attempted to Germanize their Polish subjects through the control of the school system and through industrialization, which led to the emergence of middle- and working-class strata in its territories. In the Russian-occupied lands, education was also controlled and use of the Polish language was banned. But in the Austrian-controlled lands, the old Polish nobility remained dominant and the former social system was preserved.

At the beginning of the twentieth century, the Polish lands featured an agrarian economy, with over 70% of the population living in rural areas (Kwasniewicz 1993). Poland's chance for independence came in 1917–18 when revolution destroyed the Russian Empire, and the Austro-Hungarian and German Empires collapsed after World War I. Poland declared its independence in November 1918 and raised an army under Marshal Joseph Pilsudski to establish its borders. The victorious Western allies supported the new Polish state and secured its western boundaries with German-occupied land; in the east, Poland fought a war against the new Soviet Union which ended in August 1920 with the defeat of the Red Army near Warsaw. The resulting peace treaty allowed Poland to regain much of its former eastern territory.

The Polish Republic

The Polish government immediately set about unifying the different parts of the country by enforcing the same legal, political, administrative, educational, and banking systems in all formerly occupied territories. "Poles," states Davies (1984:120), "who had lived all their lives in Russia, Prussia, or Austria had developed quite distinct habits and could not adapt to each other overnight." Nevertheless, considerable progress was made in establishing a Polish state on all fronts, except in parliamentary politics. Bickering and disagreements between the various political parties persisted. The first president was assassinated shortly after his election in 1922. Davies finds that with the officer corps of the army openly contemptuous of politicians and unwilling to submit to civilian control over military affairs, the stage was set for mutiny. And this is exactly what happened in 1926 when Pilsudski seized the government in a coup d'etat. Pilsudski did not operate as an overt dictator, allowing parliament, political parties, and limited opposition to his government to exist, but he ruled Poland in a dictatorial manner until his death in 1933. Davies (1984:126) provides the following assessment:

> Pilsudski's Poland had several redeeming features. On the surface at least, it exuded a spirit of debonair confidence. Polish cultural life saw an explosion of literary and artistic talent. Economic life, if not prosperous, was at least stable. . . . Political repression did not affect the mass of the population. There was no enforced ideology. The great Marshal was the object of much adulation and much genuine affection.
>
> Yet the system, like the Marshal himself, was seriously ill. Social distress in the countryside was acute. Unemployment in Polish industry during the Depression reached 40%. Intercommunal antagonisms and rising anti-semitism caused great anxiety. A new constitution, unveiled in April 1935, moved in the direction of intensified authoritarianism. The ills of society were being suppressed, not treated.

Poland's internal problems in building a modern state were compounded by its geographical location between the Soviet Union and Nazi Germany, both of which were antagonistic toward the Poles despite mutual nonaggression pacts. Although there had been some industrialization, Poland remained a largely rural agrarian nation in the 1930s and lacked the resources to modernize its army on the scale needed to deter the Soviets and the Germans. At the top of Polish society in the early 1930s were wealthy landowners who constituted 1% of the social structure, followed by entrepreneurs (2%), the professionals and the intelligentsia (5%), working class (17%), and agricultural laborers and peasants (74%); as late as 1938, some 72.6% of the population lived in rural areas (Davies 1984; Kwasniewicz 1993). Another analysis of social stratification in Poland in 1931 finds a somewhat larger working class (29.7%) and a smaller stratum of self-employed farmers or peasants (60.7%); even so, it is clear that agriculture was the leading occupational category (Zagorski 1978).

Table 7.1

Life Expectancy in Poland, 1931–1995

Year	Males	Female
1931–32	48.2	51.4
1948	55.6	62.5
1952–53	58.6	64.2
1955–56	61.8	67.8
1965–66	66.8	72.8
1970–72	66.8	73.8
1975–76	67.3	75.0
1980–81	66.9	75.4
1985	66.5	74.8
1989	66.7	75.5
1990	66.5	75.5
1991	66.1	75.3
1992	66.7	75.7
1993	67.4	76.0
1994	67.5	76.1
1995	67.6	76.4

SOURCE: Central Statistical Office, Polish Ministry of Health 1996.

As for life expectancy, table 7.1 shows that in 1931–32, Polish males lived an average of 48.2 years and females 51.4 years. At the same time, French males were averaging 54.7 years and French females 59.7 years. American males lived an average of 61 years and females 63.5 years. Consequently, life expectancy in Poland was not especially high. Poland had passed a health insurance law in 1920 which required all workers under a certain income level to be covered under its provisions. Employers paid 60% of the premiums and employees the other 40%.

Hospitals were obligated to provide medical care to all persons insured in this program for half price (Marrée and Groenewegen 1997). By 1938, however, only 30% of the Polish population was covered by health insurance (Sokolowska and Moskalewicz 1987). Hospitals and outpatient clinics were financed by local governments and various charitable and religious organizations also operated health care facilities. Thus, the state used private charity to supplement government-sponsored treatment. Overall, Poland lagged behind Western Europe in providing national health insurance coverage for the entire population, but the new nation was making an effort to cope with its health problems.

On 1 September 1939 Germany invaded Poland in the opening round of World War II. The Polish armed forces put up a fierce resistance against a much stronger and better equipped foe, managing to hold out for several days at Westerplatte near Danzig (now Gdańsk) and during the siege of Warsaw, and even counterattacking across the Bzura River. Poland's fate was sealed, however, when the Soviet Union invaded from the east on 17 September while the Poles were defending against the Germans in the west. American historian E. Garrison Walters (1988:167) writes:

> The Polish forces fought bravely but not well. Like the French, the Poles had not altered their military doctrine beyond the lessons learned in the static warfare of 1914–18. Polish forces lacked the mobility to respond to the rapid thrusts of armor and aircraft which were to give the world the word "Blitzkrieg." In any case, the absolute inability of the British and French to offer any meaningful assistance, direct or diversionary, together with the Soviet attack, made an early defeat inevitable. Warsaw was captured by German forces on September 27, and all large-scale combat ceased less than a week later. In the circumstances, the fact that the Poles resisted for a full month is a great tribute to their heroism and tenacity.

Altogether, some 6 million Poles out of a population of 35 million in 1939 lost their lives during World War II. They were either killed during the invasions or lost their lives as part of the resistance to the occupation, in the Warsaw Uprising against the Germans in 1944, or in mass executions. Poland's prewar Jewish population of over 3 million was virtually exterminated in concentration camps, along with millions more Jews from elsewhere in Europe. Several thousand Jews were also killed in the uprising in the Warsaw Ghetto in 1943, as the Jewish population struck back in armed revolt against the Nazis. The Nazis, in turn, totally destroyed the ghetto and, by war's end, much of Warsaw itself had been devastated. Another 2 million Poles, many of whom perished, were deported by the Soviet Union to work in labor camps in Siberia. No country suffered more human losses in proportion to its size during World War II than Poland (Davies 1984).

After the German surrender in May 1945 political and armed struggle between communists, supported by the Soviet Union, and various anti-communist groups continued in Poland for another two years. The Western allies had left Poland in the Soviet sphere of influence—provided free elections were held. But with the Polish opposition severely diminished through murders, arrests, deportations, and political maneuvering, a communist regime was established in 1948. This process was aided by the occupation of Poland by the Soviet Army, which had pushed the Germans out of Polish territory toward the end of World War II. The final peace settlement in Europe also changed the map of Poland, with the Soviet Union acquiring Poland's eastern provinces and the Poles being compensated by receiving former German lands in the west. The Poles in the east were involuntarily transferred in mass to the new western lands, while the former German population was made to leave. This forced migration was to have a significant impact on the health of the Poles in the new territories.

The Communist Period

Poland emerged from World War II as a Soviet client state with a communist government imposed over a largely Catholic population. This was an uneasy fit. Key government posts were held only by trusted Polish communists or Soviets with Polish names. The period between 1948 and 1956 (until after Stalin's death) was one of repression as further efforts were made to persecute opponents of the regime and others who lacked enthusiasm for it. Efforts were also made to collectivize farming and the Catholic Church was harassed, including by the arrest of its leading cardinal. The country was subjected to an intense process of industrialization with emphasis upon heavy industry and mining. These years, as Polish sociologist Wladyslaw Kwasniewicz (1993) points out, were particularly difficult. "The decisive influence on the course of events in Poland," states Kwasniewicz (1993:167), "was exerted by openly pro-Stalinist forces, which were taking no notice of Polish reality and attempted to shape Polish society according to ideological models imposed by the Kremlin."

Poland's traditional social order had been destroyed during World War

II and the communist takeover. The new social structure was similar to that of the other European socialist countries, with the small Communist Party elite occupying the top rung of the social ladder, followed by managers of state enterprises, the intelligentsia, technical specialists, blue-collar workers, and peasants/agricultural workers. In 1960, the largest stratum was the peasantry (over 44%) and the second largest the blue-collar workers (33.8%); by 1972, the two classes had switched positions, with blue-collar workers comprising 42.2% of the population and peasants 32.5% (Zagorski 1978). A lasting influence from the precommunist era was the strong social distinction between manual and nonmanual labor. Nonmanual work had much higher status than manual labor. Even though the social position of manual workers improved dramatically under communism, they still occupied a subordinate position in the labor force and "in everyday life even today the distinction between manual and nonmanual workers is very pronounced" (Kohn and Slomczyński 1990:39). Among manual workers, there was a further distinction

> which divides all manual workers of the nationalized economy into two classes: those who are employed in the large-scale manufacturing and extractive enterprises of the centralized economy—in steel mills, ship building, auto manufacture, coal mining—and those who are employed in secondary and supportive industries and in service—in transportation, food processing, and repair. The former we call "production workers," constitute the core of the working class; the latter, whom we call "non-production workers," constitute the periphery. In the nationalized economy of Poland in 1978, this distinction was not only descriptive of labor-market segmentation, but constituted a true class distinction. Production workers have been the main force in the immediate bargaining process with the government. Economically, production workers have been pivotal to socialist industrialization; this has been treated by the Government as a factor legitimizing the privileges given to these workers. (Kohn and Slomczyński 1990:39)

Although Poland lost most of its characteristics as a rural society at the hands of the communists and became an industrial and urban society, its peasantry retained over 30% of the population in its ranks. This is a much larger proportion of peasants than is found in most former socialist countries. Moreover, this was a free peasantry as Poland's farmers were generally able to escape collective agriculture and maintain private ownership of their plots. The decisive event in this development was an uprising in Poznań in 1956 led by students and workers. Some 74 people were killed and several were arrested. A shock wave went through the Communist Party leadership, who realized they did not have widespread popular support. Despite initially strong dissent from the Soviet premier Nikita Khrushchev, the Polish communists appointed Wladyslaw Gomulka as their leader. Gomulka was a loyal servant of the Soviet Union, yet was able to reduce state repression to one of its mildest forms in the Soviet bloc. The collectivization of agriculture was stopped and the peasants regained land taken from them, a rapprochement with the Catholic Church was begun, and Soviets serving in Polish government posts were dismissed and sent home. But aside from these measures Gomulka's regime did not have a broad program of reform and controls were tightened on the population as time went by. There were serious instances of student unrest in 1968 and, finally, in 1970, there was another workers' revolt at the Lenin Shipyard in Gdańsk. Some 45 workers were killed and Gomulka was ousted from power by the Communist Party in the aftermath of public reaction to the killings.

The new party boss, Edward Gierek, took a similar route as Gomulka. He initially appeared to be a reformer but continued repression with the same unstinting loyalty to Moscow. However, in an effort to improve living conditions and satisfy worker demands, Gierek borrowed heavily from Western banks, imported meat, controlled the prices of food at artificially low levels, and raised wages. Peasants, who had been excluded from the national health insurance system if they were private farmers, gained eligibility for state-provided health care in 1972. Prior to this time, private farmers did receive some free care from the state, such as vaccinations, treatment of contagious and "social diseases" (like tuberculosis and sexually transmitted diseases), medical care for infants until the age of one, and maternity care. In case of hospitalization, they could apply for free care if they could prove they lacked financial resources. After they received access to the full range of state health services, however, their use of such services did not significantly increase.

But Gierek's economic approach was doomed from the beginning. Substandard Polish goods were not in demand in Western markets, so investment in manufacturing was fruitless. In the meantime, Polish agriculture was increasingly unable to feed the nation. Price increases on food stuffs set off worker revolts in Warsaw and Radom in 1976; the revolts were quelled and the government responded by borrowing even more money from the West. Yet the Polish economy could not recover because its system of centralized planning and state ownership was too rigid and inefficient to be productive. American journalist Flora Lewis (1987:410) describes the situation in Polish agriculture at the time as follows:

Living standards deteriorated. Polish agriculture, once an important supplier to Europe, could not feed the country's own people. This too was largely of the regime's making. The private farmers were a good deal more productive than the collective and state farms. But the party had never really given up its aim of corralling them back into "socialized" agriculture. It could no longer use force, but it did everything else possible to discourage private farmers. The quarter of the land under state control got more than half the supplies of seed and fertilizer. Prices were skewed so that it was often cheaper for peasants to buy bread to feed their animals than to buy feed. The only tractors produced in the country were huge, heavy ones suitable for vast "socialized" tracts, but the private farmers were seldom allowed more than a few acres. So they continued, as in ages past, to rely on horses, clumsy wooden carts and inadequate plows and equipment. The regime was willing to spite the anticollectivist farmers at whatever cost to the country.

Opposition to the government in the 1970s began to grow. The influence of the church was important, which was especially evident in the 1979 visit of the Pope to Poland when millions of people turned up to greet him and hear his words. Also important was the widespread organization of unofficial trade unions, which became a large-scale workers' movement in 1980 under the banner of *Solidarnosć*, or Solidarity. The catalyst for this latter development were the labor strikes called in August 1980 when the government unexpectedly raised food prices again. Under the leadership of Lech Walesa, a former electrician at the Lenin Shipyard in Gdańsk, Solidarity demanded the right to be officially recognized as a free and independent trade union, along with a series of other demands such as better health care, promotion on the basis of talent rather than party service, the right to strike, and more meat in the shops (Stokes 1993). With the support of intellectuals, Solidarity had the power to initiate a nationwide labor strike. The government backed down and a series of agreements known as the Social Accords were signed in 1981—giving Solidarity what it wanted.

The Communist Party was in disarray. Gierek was replaced as prime minister. There was a massive decline in party membership and the gap between the party and the general population widened. As Raymond Wong (1995:309) explains: "Strong workers' movements and the autonomy of the Catholic Church provided alternative value systems to legitimize struggles against the socialist regime and specific government policies that were unfavorable to workers or perceived to aggravate inequality." Solidarity's membership reached 10 million and it was clear that the union was on a collision course with the government. In early 1980 there was a possibility of invasion by the Soviet Union to crush the rising dissent in Poland, but the Polish Communist Party made the defense minister, General Wojciech Jaruzelski, the new prime minister. Jaruzelski declared a "state of war" in December 1981 and in a well-executed and generally successful military operation arrested most of Solidarity's leaders, imposed full censorship, took control of the coal mines (after killing some striking miners), and created military courts that sentenced dissidents to prison terms (Stokes 1993).

But martial law (which was lifted in 1983) did not solve the nation's problems. The economic crisis worsened and Solidarity, though seriously weakened, continued as an underground organization. Walesa, released from prison, received the Nobel Peace Prize in 1983 and continued to conduct himself as an uncompromising public opponent of the government. Pope John Paul II, on a visit to Poland in 1987, drew millions to his sermons speaking of human rights and the benefits of multiparty politics, while granting Walesa a private audience. There were signs of some softening on the regime's part as security police responsible for the murder of a popular antigovernment Catholic priest, Jerzy Popieluszko, were given a public trial and prison sentences. Jaruzelski had come to realize that he could not ignore public opinion (Stokes 1993).

However, the economy continued to fail. Jaruzelski had made the decision to expand trade with the Soviet Union since economic constraints had been imposed by the West after martial law. "Unable to import new technology from the West," states Gale Stokes (1993:119), "and tied into the slipshod Soviet market, Polish industry became less and less able to compete." Long lines for the purchase of goods reappeared in 1988—a time characterized humorously as one in which "everyone's fondest dream was to be able to locate a roll of toilet paper" (as quoted in Stokes 1993:118). When the Soviet market collapsed in 1990, Poland was left with many obsolete industries and a huge trade deficit.

Strikes in early 1988 led to roundtable talks with the government reinstating Solidarity, and the agreement eventually reached included free multiparty elections. With Mikhail Gorbachev's policy of nonintervention in the internal affairs of the Soviet Union's Eastern European client states, open and free elections in 1989 signaled the end of communist Poland. Solidarity candidates rode a strong tide of votes support into parliament and noncommunist Tadeusz Mazowiecki became prime minister.

One of the major issues of Solidarity's campaign to improve conditions in Poland under communism was better health care. As Antonina Ostrowska (1993:44) comments: "The malfunctioning of the health system was one of the elements leading to the protest that initiated transformation in 1981." When the communists took power in the late 1940s, they installed a Soviet-style health care delivery system focused on meeting the health needs of workers. Preexisting health facilities were placed under government ownership and health care providers were made employees of the state. The Ministry of Health and Welfare was responsible for the health care of the majority of the population, but special groups like the party elite, army, police, miners, and railway workers had their own separate facilities under different state ministries (Marrée and Groenewegen 1997). Consequently, Poland, like the other former socialist countries, had a stratified hierarchy of health care facilities with privileged groups receiving special treatment which still exists today. Primary care for the general population was provided in urban polyclinics or rural health stations. The "productive" sector of core manufacturing enterprises also had its own health care system, known as industrial medicine. Large factories had their own doctors and nurses, with the largest having hospitals and health spas. These facilities were usually better equipped than the regular urban and rural polyclinics. Workers could use whichever facility (urban or industrial) they wanted.

During the first 20 years of communism, the Polish health care delivery system was neglected by the government. Priority went to the development of heavy industry and social services like health care were regarded as "nonproductive" (Millard 1984). When Gierek came to power in 1970, promised reforms included health care. However, other than some organizational changes, Poland's health system remained in a poor state, with serious shortages of supplies and modern equipment (Sheahan 1995). Andrew Nagorski (1993), for example, found that in some hospitals in the 1980s patients had to provide their own cots to sleep on and occasionally—when supplies were short—children underwent tonsillectomies without anesthesia. Until 1986 there was no choice of physicians; people were assigned to a polyclinic in their area and were supposed to be treated by whatever physician was available, but in reality people could often choose a doctor from their assigned polyclinic. After 1986 it was "officially" possible to choose one's own doctor at the health facility.

However, primary care in Poland did not have a good reputation because most of the clinics were underequipped. Many patients went directly to specialists since referrals for secondary care were not required (Marrée and Groenewegen 1997). In order to get more personalized care, many patients paid gratuities to physicians and other health care personnel which, Ostrowska (1993) argues, corrupted the system. But

Ostrowska also notes that under-the-table payments made real socialism more bearable. Private medicine existed for those who could pay out of their own pockets as some 30% of Polish physicians worked a few hours each day on a fee-for-service basis after providing state-sponsored care (Roemer 1994). Fees-for-service came in addition to the low salaries paid by the state, and sometimes this work was given a higher priority by the physicians involved. As Ostrowska (1993) points out, Polish medical doctors were encouraged to perform their duties according to some vague socialist-physician model and were not paid very well accordingly. "Living up to this model could not have been a very convincing goal," states Ostrowska (1993:44), "considering the fact that physicians in the communist system became a visibly corrupt group."

Poland did avoid the severe downturn in life expectancy for males that occurred in Russia and Hungary. Decline came, but it came later. Table 7.1 shows that life expectancy for Polish males neither fell nor rose in the mid-1960s, but remained at 66.8 years in 1965–66 and 1970–72. By 1975–76, there had actually been a small increase to 67.3 years. However, the decrease began at this point and by 1985 male life expectancy had fallen to 66.5 years. A slight recovery was made to 66.7 years in 1989, at the end of the communist period, but at this time it is clear that a downward trend is underway. For Polish women, the pattern went generally upward, except for a small decrease in 1985. Polish women lived 72.8 years on average in 1965–66 and 75.5 years in 1989.

The Postcommunist Period

After 1989, Poland began the transition to a capitalist economy and switched its trade orientation from Eastern to Western markets. But the economy was practically bankrupt after years of communist rule and the change to a free-market system was painful. Many people were disappointed at the slow rate at which improvements were coming and fearful of the loss of the security provided by socialism (guaranteed jobs, pensions, etc.). Both inflation and unemployment were high in Poland in the early 1990s. Jaruzelski, still viewing himself as a savior of Poland from a Soviet invasion through his declaration of martial law, resigned as president under pressure in 1990 (Rosenberg 1995). Walesa became Poland's first popularly elected president in December 1990. Walesa's time in office was controversial, however, as he sought increased presidential powers in a new and uncertain political system and became enmeshed in conflicts

with various political opponents. The Solidarity political coalition frag-
mented as different groups within its ranks broke off in various directions,
unable to compromise with one another (Zubeck 1993). Having won
power, Solidarity was unprepared to exercise it. The government they
inherited lacked trained personnel to operate its bureaucracies, nor did
they have an economic program on hand to transform the economy.

As for Walesa, one of his most important talents, according to Polish
political scientist Voytek Zubeck (1990), was his ability to sway working-
class crowds through impromptu speeches. "Walesa's folksy sense of
humor, avuncular pose, and manner of speech, full of working class gram-
matical idiosyncrasies and accentuated by his muted peasant–working
class accent," states Zubeck (1990:69), "built a natural bond of almost
familial acceptance between him and the crowd, and their enthusiasm
propelled him into the position of their tribune." But Walesa was not well
educated, even described by some as semiliterate; moreover, he was often
temperamental, authoritarian, and given to verbal outbursts (Zubeck
1997). As the leader of Solidarity, his outrageous statements were usually kept from public view or mediated by intellectuals who shared his
goals. Yet as president his personal traits were more open to scrutiny by
the media and the public. Walesa was elected by two-thirds of the popular vote in 1990, but only 54% of the eligible voters participated so his
support was never high and had seriously eroded by the 1995 presidential elections. Televised debates against his urbane and former communist opponent, Alexander Kwasniewski, were a disaster as Walesa
appeared rambling, incoherent, and belligerent at times (Zubeck 1997).
Nevertheless, Walesa lost the election by a narrow margin of 48.3% of
the vote versus Kwasniewski's 51.7%. As Zubeck (1997:107) explains:

> Although Eastern Europe's 1989 "Revolution" was largely bloodless, it
> devoured most of its heroes and the leaders of the Solidarity movement
> were not exempt from this fate. . . . By the 1990s most Poles viewed these
> same individuals as just another group of shifty politicians undeserving of
> their trust. This decline from exalted leader to untrustworthy politician was
> also shared by Lech Walesa, who led the Solidarity movement. Next to
> Gorbachev, Walesa was the most important leader of the revolution which
> brought down the Iron Curtain. Idolized in the 1980s for his idealistic fer-
> vor, Walesa began to be viewed in the 1990s as just another individualistic,
> ruthless and controversial politician, responsible for political chaos in
> Poland. Walesa's decline tells a great deal about the diverse and contradic-
> tory groups formerly united by anti-communist fervor who brought down
> the government, only to splinter into many factions when the revolution
> was over.

Kwasniewski's election was upsetting to many anticommunists, but this development did not signal a recommunization of Poland. Rather, Poland's leading government officials included both ex-communists and noncommunists, including members of Solidarity. The Solidarity coalition, in fact, made a strong comeback in the 1997 parliamentary elections. Earlier, in 1990, Poland had introduced economic and financial "shock therapy." At that time, wages were temporarily frozen, but the core of the program was the removal of all price controls, the phasing out of subsidies from unprofitable state enterprises, and privatization. These measures produced significant unemployment, which in 1996 still included nearly 15% of the labor force. Inadequate pensions for retirees also remain an important problem. Since 1996, reforms have been slowed. However, Poland, with a current population of 38.6 million, shows some of the strongest economic growth in Europe—despite the persistence of high inflation and unemployment. Beginning in 1994, most macroeconomic performance indicators began to markedly improve. The pace of real GDP growth has risen steadily since 1992, but reached 5.2% in 1994 and a high of 7% in 1995. Poland's living standards, however, are still 30% below those of the European Union average, and about 40 to 50% of the levels in Spain, Portugal, and Greece. Yet the country's economic transition to capitalism has been one of the most successful ones among the former socialist countries (OECD 1996). In 1997, Poland was invited to join NATO and in 1998 an invitation was forthcoming to discuss membership in the European Union. Poland is moving back into Europe's mainstream.

The extent to which Poland has westernized is particularly apparent to people from other former socialist countries. Nagorski (1993:280) reported on conditions in Przemysl, a Polish town near the Ukrainian border. He interviewed a man who had a house built by a Ukrainian construction team. This man had earned his money as a construction worker in Chicago and could pay the Ukrainians in two days what they were usually paid for an entire month's work in the Ukraine. To the Ukrainians, Poland was the West with its higher living standards, better pay, and better treatment of the individual. In Moscow, a Russian writer explained to Nagorski that the difference between Russia and Poland was that a person could cross the border from Germany into Poland and see that Poland may be poorer and dirtier—but it is still Europe. Crossing from Poland into Russia, however, a person did not get the same impression. The Russian border region seemed a different world in which time seemed to have stood still for many years. Nagorski (1993:281–82) comments:

Some Poles, Hungarians, and Czechs may still have had serious doubts about the extent of their countries' westernization, but not the Russians, Ukrainians, and others who made such voyages. In late 1991, on a flight from Warsaw to Moscow, I sat beside Boris Kharlov, a factory director from the Urals. He had just spent a week in Poland arranging to barter the engines his factory produced for Polish food shipments. We chatted about his trip and his impressions of Poland, and then I asked whether he had ever been to the West. "No, this is my first time," he replied, perfectly seriously.

Economic change has had a corresponding influence on Poland's class system. The emerging class system is not well defined. One reason is the extensive "shadow," or unofficial economy, whose activities are unreported but generate income and trade. Nevertheless, it is clear that Poland's class structure is undergoing a process of recomposition and becoming more similar to the West (Domański 1994; Kohn et al. 1997; Slomczyński 1997). Since the late 1940s, social class position in socialist Poland has been primarily determined by occupation, with education determining the status associated with a person's job to a much greater extent than income (Slomczyński and Krauze 1986). In the postcommunist period, however, income has grown in significance in influencing an individual's location in the class structure (Domański 1994). Some Polish entrepreneurs have become wealthy and opened up a large gap in income between themselves and the rest of the population. Another significant development is the rise of a new middle class which is also a major beneficiary of the introduction of capitalism. The next two strata in Polish society, the working class and the peasants, have been hit hardest by unemployment. There is a growing number of poor and homeless people as well.

As for health care delivery, little organizational change has taken place to date in the postcommunist period. The former Soviet-style system has remained largely in place, with health personnel managed and supported by the state (Marrée and Groenewegen 1997; Ostrowska 1993). The bulk of payments for service still comes directly from the central government's budget. In 1991, some 5.1% of the GDP was spent on health, which dropped to 5% in 1992 and remained stable at 4.7% for 1993–95. With the fall of communism, privatization was expected to be a major feature of health policy. But little privatization took place until the mid-1990s. Some cooperative and private clinics have existed since communist times to supplement the government system. Cooperative clinics, are medical treatment facilities organized by physicians to provide outpatient care; physicians in these facilities are paid salaries by the state but are allowed to have some private patients. Patients now have the liberty to choose any physician in Poland. There are also some private medical practices and clinics, and privatization policies have also resulted in the use of state facilities by doctors to treat patients after normal working hours. On balance, however, Poland's health care delivery system remains unchanged. Most doctors are state employees and the practice of gratuities for more personal care remains in place, but it is also understood by patients that physician salaries in state clinics are very low and gratuities are a good way to show their appreciation.

Table 7.1 shows that male life expectancy in Poland stood at 66.5 years in 1990 and declined to 66.1 years in 1991. There was an increase to 66.7 years in 1992, and in 1993 longevity rose to 67.4 years and to 67.6 years in 1995. Currently, life expectancy for Polish men is only slightly better than what it was 30 years ago. During the same period, the life expectancy for French and American men, in contrast, increased by 6.1 and 5.7 years respectively. Although Polish male longevity has shown periods of decline during the communist era, the declines have not been as severe as in Russia and Hungary; rather, the best summarization is to describe the overall pattern as one of stagnation. Polish women, on the other hand, have witnessed a general rise in life expectancy with a 1995 figure of 76.4 years, which is somewhat less than that found in the West but nevertheless is positive. Polish women in 1995 lived 3.6 years more on average that they did in 1965, compared to women from France who gained 7.1 years and from the United States who advanced 5.2 years over the same period.

POLISH MORTALITY PATTERNS

As in the other former socialist countries, the people most affected by adverse health in Poland were middle-aged working-class males, who suffered premature deaths from heart disease. According to Polish demographer Marek Okólski (1993), changes in mortality related to heart disease were largely responsible for the increase in mortality in Poland and Eastern Europe generally. Okólski finds that death rates from heart disease for Polish men between 1962 and 1988 increased 296% for the 40- to 44-year-olds, 235% for the 45- to 49-year-olds, 226% for the 50- to 54-year-olds, and 177% for ages 55 to 59. Other data show that overall male mortality rates rose from 603 deaths per 100,000 population in 1970–75 to 781 in 1987, only to decrease somewhat to 760.8

in 1992 (Marrée and Groenewegen 1997). Heart disease mortality was particularly concentrated among manual workers (Makowiec-Dabrowska 1995; Watson 1998).

Thus, for males, incidence of heart disease was rising at a time when mortality from this affliction was declining in Western countries. For Polish women, heart disease mortality rates were much lower than for men at 458.9 per 100,000 in 1992. Cancer mortality has increased in Poland, with male rates exceeding female rates in 1992 with 293.3 deaths per 100,000 persons versus 153.5. Males also led overwhelmingly in deaths from external injuries and poisonings (132.5 per 100,000 compared to 35.7 for women) and diseases of the respiratory system (62.9 versus 21.7). The most promising signs today are the decline in mortality from heart disease since the early 1990s and the increase in life expectancy which have been consistent for females and have been moving upward for males since the mid-1990s. But, when it comes to poor health, it is the middle-aged male manual worker who is most susceptible to dying prematurely. Although in decline, heart disease is still responsible for half of all deaths in Poland. Data from 1995 show, for example, that 50.4% of Polish mortality was caused by heart disease, 20.5% by cancer, and 7.5% by injuries and poisonings.

THE SOCIAL DETERMINANTS OF LIFE EXPECTANCY

As discussed earlier in this book, the major determinants of poor life expectancy in the former socialist countries are not biomedical, such as infectious disease, genetics, and the like. Poland does have serious problems with environmental pollution, especially in the mining and manufacturing areas of Silesia along the northern Czech border. The most polluted area in Poland is the central part of Katowice Province west of Cracow. In this region, residue from the mining of coal, zinc, and lead, along with metal and chemical wastes from local factories, have caused serious damage to soils, plants, and air quality (Gzyl 1997). However, as also noted earlier, environmental pollution cannot be considered the primary cause of Poland's health problems (Brown, Goble, and Kirschner 1995; Hertzman 1995). Once again, I turn to an examination of the effects of the social determinants of policy, societal stress, and health lifestyles on male mortality.

Policy

Although health care delivery in Poland has not been generally regarded as a high-quality service, medical treatment and the policy that shapes its delivery cannot be regarded as the source of early deaths from heart disease among middle-aged working-class males (Ostrowska 1997; Zatonski et al. 1998). Medical care is widely available in Poland and there are excellent cardiovascular specialists and heart disease clinics in major cities like Warsaw. The failure of Poland's health care policy is the same as that of the other former socialist countries in that the emphasis was placed on secondary prevention (or the early detection of disease by doctors in clinics and offices) and not on primary prevention (or the practice of encouraging healthy lifestyles), although there have been public health campaigns to curb smoking and alcohol consumption.

The major problem in reforming the health care delivery system has been financing. The health system has been historically underfunded and primary care practitioners—the first line of medical treatment—have usually lacked in staff, office space, supplies, and the motivation to establish long-term care programs with patients (Ostrowska 1993; Sheahan 1995). It was often easier to forward patients on to specialists. One area in which some reform has taken place, however, is primary care. The concept of a "family physician," which was missing under socialism, has been created, and general practitioners are being encouraged to adopt this approach. Another area of reform is health insurance, and an insurance system will be introduced in 1999 that will be financed by contributions from employers, employees, and tax revenues. This development is a major change for the Polish people and marks the most serious alteration to date of the former socialist system. While the health care delivery system itself is in the process of catching up with the economic, social, and political changes taking place, Poland's past and current health policies have not been the cause of the country's problems with male longevity. Rather, they have failed to contain those problems and allow Polish men to reach or extend their natural life span.

Societal Stress

The societal stress explanation maintains that macro-level stressors in the wider society—such as a failing economy, depressed living standards, structural limitations on personal aspirations, political repression, and the like—produce adverse physiological reactions within the body. These reactions, in turn, have the potential to cause ill health and premature mortality among vulnerable people. This area of research has received little attention in the former socialist countries as a possible causal factor in the downturn in longevity. However, a Polish survey (Szadkowska-Stanczyk and Hanke 1991) found that stress was considered by many people to be a particularly important risk factor for heart disease. This research, consisting of a random sample of persons living in both an urban (Wroclaw) and a rural area (Ciechanow), disclosed that a high proportion of males, but not females, admitted considerable psychological distress about low wages, marriage difficulties, and poor work conditions. The extent to which these stressors may have actually played a role in heart disease was not specified, but the study does suggest that some Poles feel stress is an important risk factor.

In general, it remains unclear whether stress per se helps induce cardiovascular problems or whether its effects are more indirect and operate through the promotion of greater drinking, smoking, neglect of diet, loss of sleep, and an inability to relax. Okólski (1993) appropriately suggests that greater research on the relationship between stress and heart disease is needed in Eastern Europe. But, until a significant body of research findings can show otherwise, the position in this book is that the role of stress is largely indirect and functions through the inducement of poor health lifestyles.

Health Lifestyles

The strongest evidence regarding the origin of Poland's mortality situation is found in unhealthy lifestyle practices. Two of the best sources of support for this conclusion come from the research of Polish sociologists Antonina Ostrowska (1997) and Janusz Bejnarowicz (1994). Using data from her own 1995 nationwide health lifestyle survey and a review of past Polish studies, Ostrowska (1997) determined that the poor state of health of Poland's population was not due to a lack of medical care. Rather, it was the unwillingness of the Polish people to adopt a healthy lifestyle. A majority of Poles took a relatively passive approach to their health and, at most, engaged in only one or two healthy lifestyle activities (such as trying to reduce stress or limiting smoking). There was an absence of personal strategies about maintaining an overall healthy lifestyle, although people were aware of the need to be generally careful about their diet, drinking, smoking, exercise, and other lifestyle practices. Moreover, a long life was not particularly valued. People wanted to enjoy themselves in the present, which promoted alcohol use. Ostrowska also found that some Poles were fatalistic in their thinking—they believed that whatever will happen will happen and there is nothing they could do to control matters. This attitude constituted a habitus (to use Pierre Bourdieu's [1984] term), or mind-set, providing an established orientation toward the world and a manner of behaving within it. In the case of Poland, maintains Ostrowska, this habitus promoted unhealthy lifestyle practices that were followed routinely and more or less unconsciously by individuals. The most common practice for maintaining one's health was visiting a physician, which Ostrowska classifies as a passive rather than active mode of conduct since the individual places his or her health in the hands of someone else (a physician) rather than actively trying to be healthy on one's own. She concludes that Poles prefer medical intervention in the case of declining health instead of opting to engage in a healthy lifestyle, and suggests that a Western-style middle class must emerge in Poland before it would be possible to popularize a comprehensive pattern of health lifestyles for people generally.

Bejnarowicz (1994) conducted an urban/rural and interregional comparison of premature mortality in Poland. He found that since the mid-1970s rural areas have had the lowest death rates from heart disease, hypertension, stroke, and most cancers. An exception was lung cancer, the incidence of which was higher in the countryside. This finding is somewhat unusual in that typically rural death rates are higher than urban ones in most countries. Rural residents usually have a lessened availability of quality medical care and a lower standard of living. It may well be, however, that the lifestyle of peasants in Poland is more conducive to male longevity at present than that of their urban counterparts—especially middle-aged blue-collar workers.

Bejnarowicz also uncovers a striking regional difference. The worst health and highest mortality rates in Poland are found in the former German territories of Pomerania (from East Prussia) and Lower Silesia (from Silesia). The German population was removed in 1945, and the land was turned over to the Poles forcibly evacuated from Poland's former eastern provinces taken by the Soviet Union. While it might be argued that the former German lands had a better-developed infrastructure in terms of roads, bridges, housing, public utilities, industrial facilities, and hospitals than the Poles left behind in the east, this was not exactly the case. The area had been heavily damaged in World War II and the Soviets had shipped virtually everything of value to the Soviet

Union—including entire factories. The Poles brought to live in this area underwent a process of severe social disintegration. They had been uprooted from their former homes and communities and brought to an area where they lacked a sense of history, tradition, culture, and community. Furthermore, this was the only part of Poland in which agriculture was successfully collectivized as the newcomer peasants were placed on state farms, instead of receiving their own plots of land. Not surprisingly, the Poles in the new territories showed much higher rates of mortality from lung cancer, heart disease, stroke, and suicide. They also exhibited a more unhealthy lifestyle in terms of significantly greater alcohol and cigarette use than their neighbors in southeast Poland. The latter region was traditionally Polish land with a rural character, strong Catholicism, low crime, private farms, and an established network of social support in the form of family, friends, community, and church. A comparison of mortality rates in 1989–90 for persons ages 45 to 64, developed by Bejnarowicz by region, with a combined measure of alcohol and cigarette consumption, shows both the lowest alcohol/cigarette consumption and the lowest mortality rates for southeast Poland. Conversely, the regions with both the highest alcohol/cigarette use and the highest mortality rates are all located in the former German lands.

Other research on alcohol consumption, smoking, and diet further illustrate the extent to which these practices affected health in Poland. Alcohol use—primarily vodka, which comprises about 70% of all alcoholic drinks consumed—increased throughout the 1960s and 1970s, but then declined at the beginning of the 1980s. Solidarity had criticized the Polish government in 1980–81 for promoting alcohol use in order to hide social problems and obtain revenue. The government responded by reducing production, rationing alcoholic beverages, and raising prices substantially. This policy was continued after martial law and only slightly liberalized in the mid-1980s, but the fact remains that alcohol use was lower in the 1980s than it was in the 1970s and mortality from cirrhosis of the liver decreased significantly at this time (Varvasovsky, Bain, and McKee 1996). In 1990–92, however, during the economic recession "shock therapy" period, there was a 35 to 40% increase in alcohol use. Alcohol consumption rose to 10 to 11 liters of pure alcohol per capita and was facilitated by the unprecedented and illegal imports of cheap alcohol to Poland when the principles of a market economy were not well defined. These imports were severely curtailed in 1993. There was also, as seen in a 1997 Center for Public Opinion Research survey, less uncertainty among the Poles about the future of their economy. The most recent figures show that alcohol consumption had declined to 8.5 liters per capita in 1998. But even though alcohol use has decreased somewhat since the early 1990s, it still remains an important health lifestyle problem in Polish society.

Cigarette smoking may, however, be a more important cause of premature mortality in Poland than alcohol abuse. About 70,000 people between the ages of 35 and 69 die each year from the effects of smoking (Brodniak 1996). Overall, smoking causes about 50% of all male deaths and 30% of all deaths from heart disease. As of 1996, some 47% of Polish men and 23% of women over the age of 16 were smokers. These figures represent a decrease of 18% for men and an increase of 4% for women since the early 1980s (Kubik et al. 1995). However, despite a decline in male smoking, cigarette consumption remains a serious health hazard with nearly half of all adult males being current smokers, and with smoking among females, especially young adult females, on the rise. Advertising campaigns by Western tobacco companies in a country that had previously lacked commercial messages in the media is believed to have contributed significantly to high cigarette consumption. The smoking of Western cigarettes became a symbol of a free world and cosmopolitan taste, especially for young adults. As Polish sociologist Wlodzimierz Brodniak (1996:1) points out: "In this country smoking is not only the largest single preventable health risk factor, it also is one of the most important elements of the Polish lifestyle." That is, for many people, smoking is a normative pattern of behavior and one fully incorporated into their lifestyle.

Under communism, the consumption of cereal products and potatoes in Poland declined while the use of meat, fat, sugar, and dairy products in the diet increased (Sekula, Babinska, and Petrova 1997). Food, especially shortages of meat, had been a major source of discontent among Polish workers, and Gierek's regime in particular had increased meat supplies with imports from abroad to meet demands (Stokes 1993). Communist governments generally attached high priority to providing an abundance of inexpensive foods for their populations to make up for material deficiencies in other areas of life and to show the superiority of communism over capitalism (Sekula et al. 1997). But these foods were not generally of high quality, nor particularly healthy. Most diets contained high fat contents with respect to meat. Fat consumption and its demonstrated relationship to heart disease is undoubtedly a major factor in the high rates of cardiovascular mortality in the former socialist countries. Since the fall of communism, price controls and government subsidies for food have been removed and food costs have correspondingly increased. As a result, consumption of dairy products, eggs, and meat has fallen as consumers have substituted less-expensive food products for more costly ones; this measure has not been effective with respect to health, however, as the per capita dietary energy declined 7% between 1988 and 1994 (Sekula et al. 1997). Changes in diet are moving in the right direction, however, as 1995 figures show a decrease in the consumption of potatoes, beef, and animal fat and increases in eating fruit and chicken along with greater use of less-harmful vegetable fat in cooking. These dietary changes may be especially important in the decline in deaths from heart disease (Zatonski et al. 1998).

Data on leisure-time exercise in Polish society are not extensive. Among the few surveys is a 1997 Center for Public Opinion Research poll showing some 7% of the Polish population reports they often exercise strenuously and regularly, while another 7% exercise quite often, and 12% exercise irregularly. Thus the Poles seem to be like their neighbors in Russia and Hungary and physical activity is uncommon. As for the other major lifestyle practices involving alcohol consumption, smoking, and diet, Polish health lifestyles are far from positive. The typical middle-aged working-class Polish male is highly likely to consume large quantities of alcohol, smoke heavily, and eat a diet rich in fat. This lifestyle appears to be the primary social determinant of an adverse situation in life expectancy for these men.

CONCLUSION

Clearly, even though the downturn in life expectancy in Poland has not been as severe as in Russia and Hungary, the situation has been more negative than positive. The principal cause of poor health does not seem to be policy—although reforms in health care delivery have been slow in coming—or societal stress, but rather health lifestyles. Ostrowska (1997) has suggested that unhealthy lifestyles are deeply ingrained in the behavior of the Polish population, and primarily among men, and that this situation is not likely to change until a new health-conscious middle class develops and establishes a comprehensive approach to healthy living which can spread across class boundaries. This has been the case in the United States, where the origin of current health lifestyles originated in the middle and upper-middle social classes and then expanded across class lines in a manner similar to that suggested by Max

Weber in his analysis of the spread of the Protestant Ethic in Western culture (Cockerham, Abel, and Lüschen 1993; Cockerham, Kunz, and Lueschen 1988).

However, a major characteristic of communism, which has emerged in this discussion of Poland and the earlier chapters on Russia and Hungary, is that its emphasis on the collective and its devaluation of the individual undermined the motivation of people to take responsibility for their own health. Responsibility was invested in the state and its client medical profession. The state, in turn, readily accepted the responsibility, advertising it as one of the major benefits of communism, but was unable or unwilling (because medical care was not a productive sector of the economy) to deliver the standard of care needed to cope with chronic diseases and other health problems. Ostrowska (1993) theorizes that special patterns of personality are created by totalitarianism as reward and punishment teach individuals what to achieve and what to avoid. In the former socialist countries, incentives to practice a healthy lifestyle were generally lacking and the barriers to enacting such a lifestyle were considerable, given the quality of food available, the normative standards of heavy drinking and smoking among adult males, and the lack of interest in leisure-time exercise. Health was a political benefit of the communist social system, not a personal responsibility, and people generally reacted accordingly with little or no effort to engage in healthy lifestyles.

Ostrowska suggests that Poland is not ready for a health reform that would require personal expense and responsibility. People have been too dependent on the state and have come to view former state benefits as a right. The loss of this right could cause serious problems for the politicians responsible. "In a country where democracy is not yet stable," states Ostrowska (1993:46), "and where health is a well-established political value, the effect of all the problems described may have profound consequences for both political stability and the health of society." At present, the health situation in Poland does not seem likely to undergo any dramatic change in the near future, although changes are unavoidable in the long term as the nation copes with the transition out of communism and seeks to improve the health of the population.

Chapter 8

The Czech Republic and Slovakia

The Czech Republic and Slovakia have the distinction of being the only former socialist countries to have reversed the downturn in life expectancy. Beginning in the mid-1960s, longevity declined among males in the former Czechoslovakia—as in most of the Soviet bloc—only to turn upward in the mid-1980s. Consequently, the Czech and Slovak experience contains important clues about reversing rising mortality in the region. The reasons for this turnaround are the focus of this chapter. I begin with an examination of the relationship between health and social change in Czechoslovakia over the past century until 1993 when the Czech Republic and Slovakia separated. At that point, each country and its social determinants of life expectancy are discussed independently.

HEALTH AND SOCIAL CHANGE IN THE FORMER CZECHOSLOVAKIA

The current Czech Republic is composed of Bohemia and Moravia, along with part of Silesia. This territory existed as either one state or a confederation of states as early as the Middle Ages. Slovakia, on its part, belonged to the Kingdom of Hungary from around 1000 to 1918. When most of Hungary was occupied by the Turks in the sixteenth and seven-

This chapter was written with the assistance of Hana Janečková, Ph.D., School of Public Health, Postgraduate Medical School, Prague, Czech Republic.

teenth centuries, the Slovak lands became the temporary center of the surviving Hungarian state. Although Hungary regained its former territory in 1699 under the Habsburgs and reestablished Budapest as its capital, Hungarian and Slovak history remained closely connected until the end of World War I (Kirschbaum 1995). A hundred years ago, both the Czech and Slovak territories were part of the Austro-Hungarian Empire under the rule of the Habsburg emperor Franz Josef. Slovakia remained under Hungarian administration with a largely agricultural economy, since the government in Budapest did not support large-scale industrial development in the region. A major exception, however, was the mining of gold, silver, copper, and iron, along with some textile manufacturing. By 1900, the Slovak social structure consisted of a small upper class of large landowners or magnates (less than 1% of the population), the majority of whom were members of the Hungarian nobility; a small middle class of merchants, shopkeepers, and office workers (less than 7%); a working class (25%), primarily miners and artisans (gold and silversmiths); and a large peasant class (68%), of whom about 80% owned the small plots of land they farmed (Kirschbaum 1995). The average plot was less than 6 hectares or 14.8 acres.

While Hungary remained the agricultural breadbasket of the empire, the Czech lands were transformed into one of the leading industrial areas of central Europe. Sugar refining, ironworks, coal mining, beer brewing, and the manufacture of chemicals, glass, machine tools, and textiles were the major industries. A system of railroads was constructed to facilitate the transport of goods and raw materials. This industrialization came at a cost, however, because environmental pollution was common in these areas early in the twentieth century. The Czech social structure differed from that of Slovakia, as well as Russia and the other present-day Eastern European countries, by ceasing to be predominately agrarian soon after 1900 (Musil 1995). The Czech lands, in fact, were unique among the former socialist countries in that the largest precommunist social stratum was the working class, not the peasants (Lovenduski and Woodall 1987). By World War I, the proportion of the population working in agriculture (31%) had fallen below that of the working class (33%); in the process, the Czech lands had become the industrial base of Austria-Hungary—containing some two-thirds of the empire's industrial capability (Kučera and Pavlík 1995). Moreover, a sizable middle class had developed. The Czechs were well on the way to becoming a modern, developed society. With the collapse of Austria-Hungary at the end of World War I, they declared themselves an independent state on 28 October 1918 and were joined two days later by Slovakia.

The Czechs and Slovaks were linked together by a common literary language, a similar spoken language and culture, and geographical proximity. The Slovaks had sought to escape Hungarian domination and a partnership with the Czechs seemed reasonable to many on both sides. Earlier, in 1915, Tamás G. Masaryk, the first elected president of the new nation, had established a Czechoslovak government-in-exile in Paris. This entity provided a basis for Czech and Slovak political cooperation in their respective efforts at obtaining statehood. At the Paris Peace Conference in 1918, Czechoslovakia's previous declaration of independence with Slovakia as its partner was confirmed by the Western allies and the new nation was formally established.

Precommunist Czechoslovakia

Czechoslovakia began its existence, however, with serious ethnic divisions: some 31% of the population in the Czech lands were German and 22% in the Slovak lands were Hungarian; large numbers of Jews, Poles, Ruthenians (Carpathian Russians), Ukrainians, and Russians were also residents, and only some 65% of the entire population considered themselves to be Czechoslovak (Kučera and Pavlík 1995). In addition, Slovakia lacked a large metropolitan area, and approximately 16% of its population was illiterate in 1921. Yet the Czech leaders felt they needed Slovakia to create a viable state, and the linking of the Slovaks with the Czechs brought the Slovaks independence from Hungary, cultural autonomy, and the opportunity for improved social and economic conditions (Kirschbaum 1995; Průcha 1995). The Slovaks, according to Canadian historian Stanislav Kirschbaum (1995:158), expected that Czechoslovakia "would not only give them every opportunity to develop economically, socially, and politically, but that it, unlike Hungary, also would allow them to participate fully and equally in governing the state." The latter did not happen to the satisfaction of the Slovaks. As Czech historian Václav Průcha (1995:42) points out, "the dynamism of the Slovak national movement gradually came into conflict with the prevailing state ideology which did not recognize the independent identity of the Slovak nation, viewing it as a mere branch of Czechoslovakia."

Other difficulties between the Czechs and Slovaks were economic. The Czechs were not only industrially advanced, but Czech agriculture was also more productive in relation to the amount of land under culti-vation. The Slovak lands were more mountainous and the soil and cli-mate less favorable to crop production. Slovak industry was slow to develop because much of the industrial infrastructure was owned by Hungarians and taken back to that country. Overall, the Slovak econo-my was estimated in the 1920s to be 30 to 70 years behind that of the Czechs. This disparity put the Slovaks in the position of being the Czech's junior partner rather than their equal in economic matters. As Průcha (1995:42) explains:

> In the economic sphere, grave problems arose in Slovakia after 1918. The adjustment of the Slovak economy to the new situation was far from easy under the conditions of the competitive prevalence of Czech capital, and it is fully understandable that numerous economic and social disorders should have arisen. Until 1938, Slovakia . . . was little more than an agrar-ian appendage of the Czech Lands, supplying it with raw materials. In trade with the Czech Lands, Slovakia exported items like cereals, magne-site, crude oil, timber, paper, and building materials. On the other hand, Slovakia depended on Czech exports of, among other things, coal, coke, metals, engineering products, chemicals, glass, porcelain, and beer. Generally, as an outlet of Czech goods, Slovakia ranked fourth or fifth, after Germany, Austria, Yugoslavia, and perhaps Britain.

In the 1920s and 1930s, Czech industry expanded and the country became one of the leading industrial centers in Europe. The social struc-ture changed accordingly. A study of Czechoslovakia's class system in 1930 showed that the population of 14 million people could be divided into five classes: (1) an upper class of capitalists, intellectuals, and top government officials (0.9%); (2) an upper-middle class of the same type of people as the upper class, but much less wealthy and powerful (5.8%); (3) a lower-middle class of merchants, some farmers, teachers, and small entrepreneurs (29.6%); (4) an upper-lower class of skilled industrial workers, white-collar workers, small shopkeepers, and some peasants (24.9%); and (5) a lower-lower class of semiskilled and unskilled industrial and agricultural workers (38.8%) (Lovenduski and Woodall 1987). It is clear that by the 1930s Czechoslovakia was well on the way to developing a much more complex and modern system of social stratification than elsewhere in the region at that time. The soci-ety was beginning to resemble its Western counterparts much more so than its Eastern neighbors, with a large middle class, a high proportion of industrial workers spread through the lower-middle and lower classes on the basis of their occupational skill levels, and the lack of a huge peasant class dwarfing the rest of society with their numbers.

Czechoslovakia had a highly regarded health care system that originated under the Austro-Hungarian monarchy. In 1870 a law on public health measures was adopted that established a program to prevent infectious diseases. In 1888 a social insurance law introduced a system of public health insurance in Austria and the Czech lands similar to that established earlier in 1883 by Bismarck in Germany. Blue-collar workers had an obligatory fee deducted from their wages to pay for their care and that of their families. Between the two world wars, Czechoslovakia belonged to the most developed countries of Europe, and its system of health care delivery was continued after the breakup of Austria-Hungary.

Table 8.1 shows male life expectancy for the Czech lands rose from 47 years in 1920–22 to 56.5 years in 1937; female life expectancy rose from 50.8 years to 60.5 years. For the same period, male longevity in the Slovak lands rose from 43.4 years to 51.8 years and for females the increase was from 45.1 to 54.7 years. By 1937, Czech men and women lived, on average, about 5 more years than Slovak men and women. This difference was largely due to higher infant and child mortality, along with lower levels of hygiene and medical care (Kučera and Pavlík 1995). Czech men in 1937 also had a slightly longer life expectancy (56.5 years) than French men (56.1 years), but were outlived by American males (58 years). Czech women lived 60.5 years in 1937 compared to 62.1 years for French and 62.4 years for American females. Consequently, in the late 1930s, the Czech lands in Czechoslovakia reflected levels of life expectancy, social stratification, and industrialization very similar to those of the West. Except for its geographical location in the heart of Central Europe, Czechoslovakia was essentially a Western European country with a relatively high standard of living in its western areas and a culture reflecting a strong literary and artistic heritage.

However, Czechoslovakia's independence ended in 1938 after the Munich Agreement, signifying the capitulation of Great Britain and France to Adolf Hitler's demand for the return of the Sudetenland to Germany. The Sudetenland, Czechoslovakia's western border region, was primarily inhabited by ethnic Germans. The Czechoslovak government was prepared to defend its border with its army; but, up against the far superior military force of Nazi Germany, abandoned by its allies, and internationally isolated, the Sudetenland was turned over to the Third Reich. Poland acquired some Czech territory in the north and Hungary took part of southern and southeastern Slovakia. Following a policy of appeasement, Britain and France hoped to avert war with Germany by allowing the Nazis to acquire what they wanted. Hitler had promised to respect the remaining Czechoslovak territory, but in 1939 Slovakia declared itself an independent state and a German ally, while the Czech lands were occupied by the German army, and Bohemia and Moravia were incorporated into the Reich as protectorates. The entire Czechoslovak territory was liberated by Soviet and American armies in May 1945.

Table 8.1

Life Expectancy in the Czech and Slovak Lands, 1920–1989

Year	Czechs		Slovaks	
	Males	Females	Males	Females
1920–22	47.0	50.8	43.4	45.1
1929–32	53.7	57.5	48.9	50.9
1937	56.5	60.5	51.8	54.7
1949–51	62.2	67.0	59.0	62.4
1960	67.6	73.4	—	—
1965	67.2	73.4	—	—
1970	66.1	73.1	66.7	72.9
1975	67.0	73.9	—	—
1980	66.8	73.9	66.8	74.2
1985	66.5	74.7	66.9	74.7
1989	68.1	75.4	67.0	75.6

SOURCES: Institute of Health Information and Statistics of the Czech Republic 1997; Kučera and Pavlík 1995; WHO Liaison Office, Slovak Republic 1998.

The Americans withdrew according to the terms of the Yalta Agreement between Stalin and the Western allies, which placed Czechoslovakia in the Soviet sphere of postwar influence. The Sudetenland was restored to Czechoslovakia and the German population deported to Germany, but the underdeveloped Ruthenian or Carpathian Russian area in the east was annexed by the Soviet Union. Slovakia regained the territory taken by Hungary in the late 1930s and many Hungarians were sent back to their homeland. Slovakia's desire to remain independent was unacceptable to the Soviets and the Slovaks once again were joined with the Czechs in a restoration of the prewar state (Kirschbaum 1995). Although a democratic, multiparty government was initially established, Communist Party members held many key bureaucratic positions and maneuvered for more power until overtly seizing control in 1948. In the Czech lands, the communists had considerable popular support in the late 1940s but this was not the case in Slovakia. Many Czechs, however, were bitter about what they felt was a betrayal of Czechoslovakia by the British and the French in 1938, and supportive of the Soviet Union for having nothing to do with the Munich Agreement and for its role in driving the Germans out (Lewis 1987). The communists took advantage of their popular appeal to remove Czechoslovakia from the ranks of capitalist societies.

The Communist Period

Once in total control of the country, the communists imposed a Stalinist-type regime with political repression and terrorism, executions of opponents, the establishment of labor camps for prisoners, curtailment of religion, and the confiscation of private property. The forced industrialization in Slovakia was also accelerated by the government as part of a continuing effort to raise the economic level and exploit the availability of raw materials. Funds and other resources to modernize Slovakia were often transferred from the Czech lands. Although the economic growth of the country went into decline after 1975, Průcha (1995) observes that the planned rate of growth continued to be higher in Slovakia than in the Czech lands. Among younger workers, differences in skills and qualifications between the two populations were erased over time. According to Průcha (1995:75):

> There is no doubt that in the whole postwar period economic development up to 1989 exhibited a greater dynamism in Slovakia than in the Czech Lands. However critical our attitude to the economic development of the country under the communist regime may be, and even though great reservations about the method of industrialization of Slovakia may be voiced, the reduction of economic and social differences between the two parts of the country in the course of several decades is an undisputed fact, which was also reflected in the social consciousness of that time. Public opinion polls undertaken in the 1970s and 1980s and also in the postcommunist period show that the population of Slovakia judged postwar economic and social developments much more favorably than the Czechs, and that until the end of 1989 the Slovaks were more optimistic about the future prospects of the country.

The process of change also altered the social structure along Soviet lines. The main instruments of destratification were government ownership of industry, redistribution of land, the collectivization of agriculture, and the abolition of private property. A drastic monetary reform wiped out the savings of the former middle and upper classes. Moreover, the children of peasants and industrial workers were given significantly higher priority in admissions to universities and technical training. By 1975, the new class system consisted of the party elite (2%); nonmanual workers, namely members of the intelligentsia, industrial managers, and technical specialists (28%); manual workers (61%); and peasants (9%). Besides the elimination of capitalists and the demotion of the formerly privileged, large numbers of peasants were moved into the working class (Lovenduski and Woodall 1987; Wong 1995). Self-employment in farming and elsewhere was practically nonexistent.

Repressive communist policies became increasingly unpopular. There were expressions of the need for reform after the death of Stalin and the revelation of many of his abuses. The Czechoslovak economy was also failing under centralized planning and government controls. Food shortages were common because of the low yields of crops from collective farms, and the Slovaks were unhappy with their loss of national autonomy. During the 1960s, the demand for change, both outside and even within the Czechoslovak Communist Party, became more acute. In 1968 there was a liberalization of government policies—the so-called "Prague Spring"—after a change of government leadership brought reformer Alexander Dubček to power. This was a short-lived attempt to build "socialism with a human face," but the reforms were crushed and Dubček was ousted when Soviet military forces and some Warsaw Pact members (Bulgaria, East Germany, Hungary, and Poland) occupied the country in August 1968. The only reform that lasted was the division of the Czech and Slovak lands into separate socialist republics under the administration of the central government in Prague.

Stalinist-style repression returned once more. In an effort to win support among the populace, the Czechoslovak government spent its cash reserves on costly Western consumer goods and made them available in the shops; however, once this artificial improvement in living standards could no longer be sustained, the economy worsened. Widespread discontent, especially among younger adults, along with poor economic conditions; Gorbachev's policy of self-determination for Eastern Europe; the fall of the Berlin Wall, the announcement of free, multiparty elections in Poland, and, finally, the spark that mobilized the population against the regime—the violent police suppression of a student protest in November 1989—resulted in large public demonstrations in Prague and elsewhere that led to the resignation of the communist government (Pryce-Jones 1995; Stokes 1993). The relative ease with which communism fell earned the title of the "velvet revolution" for the activities producing the final outcome. A notable difference between events in Czechoslovakia, as compared to Hungary and Poland, was that the masses, especially students, played a much larger role in bringing down the government (Holmes 1997). In Poland, the workers were the major catalyst for change, whereas in Hungary it was reformers within the Communist Party.

Under the communists, the Czechoslovak health care delivery system had been strictly modeled after the Soviet system described in earlier chapters. This meant that health care was financed out of the government's central budget, health workers were paid a salary, and services were provided for free, at least in theory. But patients typically paid gratuities if they wanted any advantage as elsewhere in the Soviet bloc. The shortage of some medical services and drugs was the main reason. Social inequality in the access to health services existed because of the favoritism of those in political power. A typical feature of the Czechoslovak system was its centralization and hierarchic organizational structure. Institutes of National Health at regional and district levels were responsible for all services in their area and employed the health care workers providing these services (Marrée and Groenewegen 1997). Health workers were controlled professionally by the Ministry of Health, administratively by the Ministry of Interior, and politically by the Communist Party. Furthermore, since 1968, both Czechs and Slovaks had their own ministries of health which regulated health care in their respective parts of the country; both systems were virtually identical. Hospital budgets were granted by the state. The budgets were determined historically and politically, according to the year's plan. Patients tended to have relatively long hospital stays since any money left at the end of the year had to be returned to the government. Therefore, hospitals had no incentives to be cost-effective and typically tried to spend their entire budget; additionally, morale was usually not high among physicians, who were paid low salaries and sought supplements to their income from patients (Raffel and Raffel 1992).

Although the Czechoslovak health system did not enjoy a high reputation for quality and motivation in providing patient care, life expectancy followed a more positive pattern than seen elsewhere in the former socialist countries. As seen in table 8.1, life expectancy for Czech men in 1965 was 67.2 years, which was below the 1960 level of 67.6 years. For 1970, table 8.1 shows a further drop in Czech male life expectancy to 66.1 years. In 1975, a slight rise to 67 years had taken place, but then a downturn occurred for 1980 (66.8 years) and 1985 (66.5 years). At this point in the mid-1980s, Czech males reflect the same pattern of rising mortality seen in the Soviet bloc generally. However, by 1989, the last year of communism, life expectancy had reached 68.1 years. This figure represents a gain of 1.6 years in Czech male longevity for a four-year period, which is highly unusual given the typical pattern in the socialist countries at this time. For Czech women, table 8.1 shows a relatively consistent, but undramatic, increase in life expectancy from 73.4 years in 1960 to 75.4 years in 1989.

Data for Slovakia in table 8.1 are incomplete, but the available figures show that Slovak male life expectancy rose from 59 years in 1949–51 to 66.7 years in 1970. Consequently, by 1970, Slovak males had overtaken their Czech counterparts in longevity with an average of 66.7 years versus the Czech average of 66.1 years. In 1980, both Czech and Slovak men lived an average of 66.8 years. By 1985, Slovak males once again outlived males in the Czech lands (66.9 years versus 66.5 years), but in 1989 the situation was reversed with the Slovaks showing 67 years compared to 68.1 years for the Czechs. Slovak women, on the other hand, bypassed the Czech women in 1980 with 74.2 years versus 73.9 years. At the end of communist domination in 1989, Slovak women lived 75.6 years on average in comparison to 75.4 years for Czech women.

The overall pattern of life expectancy during the communist period, therefore, consisted of the following trends: (1) male life expectancy declined from the mid-1960s to the mid-1980s when it began a recovery; (2) female life expectancy generally increased, but the rise was not striking in comparison to the West; and (3) by the 1980s the Slovaks and Czechs had relatively equal life spans. The Slovak lands, however, had been a major beneficiary of increased investment from Prague. Although development took place at a significantly lower level than that of the West it nonetheless represented a major advance in a relatively backward and underdeveloped region. Benefits included a greater share of the national income which translated into a standard of living much lower than in the West but certainly higher than what had been available previously. This improvement most likely promoted longer lives since it meant a better quality of life. But it needs to be kept in mind that while the Slovaks were able to overtake the Czechs in longevity, male life expectancy in the Czech lands was decreasing for most of the communist period and female longevity was essentially stagnating. As Czech sociologists Hana Janečková and Helena Hniličová (1992:143) explain: "If we should evaluate the health status of people in Czechoslovakia up to the present time, we are obliged to conclude that it is not good." The health care delivery system mirrored the Soviet version and focused on controlling infectious disease, requiring mandatory immunizations, and reducing infant mortality, but it was unprepared to effectively handle chronic illnesses. As elsewhere in the former socialist countries, the persons most likely to succumb to an early death were middle-aged working-class males (Carlson and Rychtaříková 1996). But it is true that male life expectancy improved in the last four years of the communist regime and an examination of the postcommunist period is needed to determine whether this trend is the beginning of a general reversal of rising male mortality, or whether it results from the accumulated effects of the prior deaths of the most vulnerable men.

The end of the communist period also meant the end of Czechoslovakia, as a fully free and democratic governmental system had to allow the Slovaks to consider independence. Although the Czechs were willing to submerge their national identity in favor of a broader Czechoslovakian nationality, the Slovaks were not. After considerable maneuvering in the political uncertainty of the initial postcommunist period, including elections and debates on a constitution, Slovak leaders opted for independence and were supported by a majority of the population (Kirschbaum 1995; Wolchik 1995; Zák 1995). As Czech sociologist Jiří Musil (1995:7) explains, "the Czech and Slovak elites did not find sufficient creativity, tolerance and strength to master the new situation which emerged after the collapse of communism and at a time when both societies had become structurally rather similar." Over the course of Czechoslovakia's history, there had been a gradual equalization in social structure, educational level, and standard of living, and it is paradoxical that the two populations split when they were more similar than ever before (Kučera and Pavlík 1995; Kirschbaum 1995; Musil 1995; Průcha 1995). The Slovaks simply wanted autonomy and their own national identity, and no longer desired to continue in what they perceived as the status of a junior partner within a postcommunist federation.

THE CZECH REPUBLIC

The new Czech Republic came into existence on 1 January 1993. Václav Havel, a former dissident and well-known playwright and author, served as the first president, with Václav Klaus as the prime minister. Under their leadership, the Czechs, like the Poles, continued the "shock thera-py" approach to economic change begun in 1990–91 by removing price controls, ending subsidies to inefficient state enterprises, and promoting privatization. By 1996 privatization was essentially complete, with 80% of all state property transferred to private ownership. Though in 1998 privatization of some strategically important enterprises like banks, coal mines, and energy companies has not been completed, and some privati-zation projects have failed, in general privatization has been a success. In the meantime, the former communist system of central planning and pro-duction quotas had been completely abandoned. The GDP increased by 2.6% in 1994, 4.8% in 1995, and 3.9% in 1996, but only 1% in 1997. Unemployment was also low for Europe, standing at 2.9% of the work-force in 1995, but since then has increased to 4.9% in 1997 and 5.6% in 1998. Nevertheless, by the mid-1990s, the Czech economy had begun a recovery, and the Czech Republic, with a 1996 population of 10.3 million people, joined Hungary and Poland as new invitees to NATO in 1997, and in discussions on membership in the European Union in 1998. The Slovak Republic awaits similar invitations.

Change in the economic system from socialism to capitalism is bring-ing a corresponding change in the class structure. As in the other former socialist countries, the shape of the new system of social stratification is still emerging with managers, supervisors, and technical specialists show-ing material gain, and manual workers emerging as the most economi-cally depressed group (Slomczyński and Shabad 1997). A survey of self-classifications of class membership conducted by the Institute of Sociology of the Czech Academy of Sciences and the STEM polling agency between 1991 and 1997 showed a decline in the percentage of persons who considered themselves middle class and a small rise in self-rankings in the lower class. In 1991, some 0.4% of the Czech respondents ranked themselves lower class; by 1997, this figure had risen to 2.5%. The proportion of persons ranking themselves in the working class declined during that same period from 38.7 to 33.8%. The lower-middle class self-ratings rose from 17.9% in 1991 to 25.7% in 1996, but decreased to 23.4% in 1997. The proportion viewing themselves as mid-dle class rose from 34.6% in 1991 to a high of 46.2% in 1995; in 1997, however, only some 31.9% ranked themselves as middle class. Taken together, the results for the lower-middle and middle classes suggest that the proportion of Czechs who think of themselves as generally middle class is declining. This development reflects a growing feeling on the part of physicians, teachers, and academics who believe their status and low wages do not reflect middle-class membership. So, despite the fact that the economy is improving and a capitalist middle class is appearing, increasing numbers of professional people sense they are moving downward. As for the upper-middle and upper classes, the percentage of self-rankings increased from 8.4 to 9.2% between 1991 and 1997.

Table 8.2

Life Expectancy in the Czech Republic, 1990–1996

Year	Males	Female
1990	67.6	75.4
1991	68.2	75.7
1992	68.5	76.1
1993	69.3	76.4
1994	69.5	76.6
1995	70.0	76.9
1996	70.4	77.3

SOURCE: Institute of Health Information and Statistics of the Czech Republic 1997.

While the Czech class structure remains fluid, there are stable signs that health is improving. Table 8.2 shows that in 1990, the year following the end of communism, male longevity was 67.6 years, which was a decline from 68.1 years in 1989 (see table 8.1). However, after this one-year decrease, life expectancy rose from 68.2 years in 1991 to a high of 70.4 years in 1996. This is the longest male life expectancy recorded in the former socialist countries, either before, during, or after communism. Life expectancy for Czech females, as shown in tables 8.1 and 8.2, has moved out of the stagnation of the 1960s and late 1970s to consistently higher levels. Table 8.2 shows, for example, that female life expectancy in 1990 was 75.4 years and by 1996 had reached a high of 77.3 years. Does this mean that the rise in mortality in the Czech Republic has been reversed? The best evidence suggests that this is indeed the case (Carlson and Rychtaříková 1996; Rychtaříková 1996). The upturn in life expectancy began in 1985 (see table 8.1) under communism when male longevity was 66.5 years and has increased consistently since then, except for a one-year drop in 1990 (see table 8.2) in the immediate aftermath of communism's collapse, which may be due to statistical error. The 55–79 age-group is most responsible for this improvement. As Czech demographer Jitka Rychtaříková (1996:3) explains:

Recently observed favorable changes in adult and elderly mortality mean more than a simple lengthening of life expectancy at birth. It is a qualitative turning point in mortality trends of the Czech Republic because until the mid eighties, mortality at ages 40 and over was deteriorating and later remained practically stationary. The high mortality at age 40+ [was] "responsible" for the overall bad placement of the Czech Republic among developed countries. The new reverse signifies the hope of a debut of the last stage of an epidemiological transition in the Czech Republic, i.e. decrease of mortality from degenerative diseases. In fact mortality started decreasing since the end of the eighties (before political changes . . .). Hence, the period of transition accompanied by political, economic, social, and behavioral transformation does not negatively influence the process of the decline already initiated. Despite the new phenomenon of unemployment, complete changes of the health care system, appearance of homeless people etc., the decline in mortality had continued.

Table 8.3

Mortality Rates for Selected Major Causes of Death per 100,000 Males, Czech Republic, 1960–1995

Causes of Death	1960	1965	1970	1975	1983	1990	1995
Cancer	273.6	318.4	329.1	367.8	349.6	361.1	345.1
Diseases of the circulatory system	599.5	681.6	795.0	785.9	871.5	834.1	708.0
Diseases of the respiratory system	131.6	152.1	184.0	149.7	124.9	81.4	62.4
Diseases of the digestive system	49.4	58.5	63.3	63.8	65.4	67.6	53.5
Traffic accidents	20.2	23.1	32.3	25.2	17.0	19.4	23.1
Suicide	40.8	39.9	43.8	37.5	33.4	30.7	25.7

SOURCE: Institute of Health Information and Statistics of the Czech Republic 1997.

Further evidence to support the claim that the Czech Republic has escaped its mortality crisis comes from cause-of-death data. Table 8.3 shows that mortality from heart disease, the leading cause of death, rose from 599.5 per 100,000 in 1960 to a high of 871.5 in 1983 and subsequently declined to 708 in 1995. Deaths from cancer also rose from 273.6 in 1960 to 367.8 in 1975. Deaths from diseases of the respiratory system likewise increased until 1970 when they stood at 184, but in 1995 had diminished to 62.4. Deaths from diseases of the digestive system have fallen since 1990, and suicide since 1970. Traffic accidents, however, increased with the onset of capitalism and the improved availability of automobiles.

Table 8.4 shows mortality rates for females for the same period. Deaths from heart disease for females increased from 502 per 100,000 in 1960 to a high of 569.3 in 1983 and fell to 454.9 by 1995. Cancer mortality rose form 181.3 per 100,000 in 1960 to 191.6 in 1990 and stood at 191.3 in 1995; deaths from cancer for women, therefore, appear to have stabilized but not decreased. Mortality from breast and lung cancer have been largely responsible for keeping these rates at their current level. Otherwise, deaths from diseases of the respiratory and digestive systems and suicide have decreased, while traffic mortality has risen but remains well below that for males.

Table 8.4

Mortality Rates for Selected Major Causes of Death per 100,000 Females, Czech Republic, 1960–1995

Causes of Death	1960	1965	1970	1975	1983	1990	1995
Cancer	181.3	187.7	183.4	173.2	189.7	191.6	191.3
Diseases of the circulatory system	502.0	498.9	545.8	532.8	569.3	519.6	454.9
Diseases of the respiratory system	71.5	70.5	70.9	67.3	57.3	29.7	31.5
Diseases of the digestive system	35.9	38.8	34.8	37.8	33.4	29.6	26.2
Traffic accidents	4.5	5.9	10.7	8.7	5.9	5.8	8.1
Suicide	17.4	15.2	15.4	13.1	10.1	9.6	7.4

SOURCE: Institute of Health Information and Statistics of the Czech Republic 1997.

In general, the Czech Republic has shown a vast improvement in its health profile in recent years. This situation has occurred despite the fact that the country is one of the heaviest polluters of air in Europe, with the major emissions coming from thermal power stations, mining, chemical industries, and automobiles (Hertzman 1995). Northern Bohemia may, in fact, contain some of the most environmentally damaged land in Europe (Janečková and Hniličová 1992). Besides the air, the ground and water have been seriously affected. Yet it is clear, as previously discussed, that pollution, while bad, has not produced a health crisis or caused the previous or current mortality problems (Hertzman 1995; Kliment et al. 1997; Peters et al. 1996). I therefore turn to the three primary social determinants of policy, societal stress, and health lifestyles.

Policy

The Czech Republic has taken an aggressive posture toward changing its health care system similar to its approach in altering the economy (Heitlinger 1993; Massaro, Nemec, and Kalman 1994). With the end of communism, health care became a major priority and health expenditures increased from 5.19% of the GDP in 1990 to 7.10% in 1994 and 6.77% in 1996. Free choices of doctors and hospitals were also allowed; patients were given direct access to medical specialists without having to go through general practitioners; and, by 1993, over 40% of all physicians—some 14,000 doctors—had made the transition to private practice (Massaro et al. 1994; Marrée and Groenewegen 1997). By 1996, nearly 60% of physicians worked in the private sector. The remaining physicians are state employees, usually of state hospitals.

Another new development is the formation of an independent health insurance company created in 1992. This company, the General Health Insurance Company (GHIC), is a nonprofit, nongovernmental organization controlled by a board consisting of 30 members representing the state, providers, and consumers. An annual report and insurance plan must be approved by the parliament yearly. The same type of control is applied to all insurance companies in the Czech Republic. The GHIC collects premiums from the insured and pays providers directly. Employers pay 9% of an employee's wages and the employee pays an additional 4.5%. Self-employed persons pay 13.5% of their net profits subject to a limitation or cap. Only the worker is insured; family members must be insured through their own place of employment or pay costs out of pocket. The government is responsible for premiums for children, students, retirees, the military, disabled persons, and the unemployed. The GHIC insures about 76% of the population; the remainder are covered by various other health insurance companies established originally for various groups of workers and subject to the same regulations.

Physicians in private practice are paid on a fee-for-service basis, with the exception of general practitioners, who are paid on either a per capita or fee-for-service basis. The doctors employed by the state, most of whom work in hospitals, receive a salary. Hospital privatization has not generally been possible because banks have refused to loan the large amounts of money required to buy these facilities from the state. There are just a few private hospitals belonging to the Catholic Church or private companies. Most hospitals remain state-owned and funded out of the central budget and fee-for-service payments from insurance companies. Instead of being given global budgets from the state in the future, hospitals will be paid by the state only for services rendered according to a Diagnostic-Related Groups (DRG) fee schedule. Many hospitals are in financial trouble because of the rising costs of drugs, medical services, and utilities, and low state budget allocations. The income from insurance companies is not sufficient to cover all hospital costs. The Czech Republic, in contrast to the countries discussed thus far—Russia, Hungary, and Poland—has a postcommunist health care delivery system more similar to those of Western Europe and many of the same problems with respect to financing and cost-effectiveness.

Nevertheless, can it be claimed that the policy decisions leading to a more Western-style health care delivery system are primarily responsible for improved mortality? The answer is no. The transformation of the health care system from the centralized Soviet-style model to the liberal model of public and private mix based on national health insurance and free choice of services is not primarily responsible for the health improvement. But it enabled many positive changes to occur. Large investments in modern technology improved the equipment and thus the diagnostic and therapeutic capabilities of Czech hospitals and private practices, along with the widespread availability of new drugs in the Czech market and improved access to new knowledge and skills available in the West. While these changes undoubtedly contributed to the rise in life expectancy, the trend toward longer male longevity actually began during late communism (1985–89) under the former socialist health care system with its poor record in containing chronic illnesses. Moreover, improvements in life expectancy are most pronounced among middle-aged males who have less contact with the health care system than any other group (Carlson and Rychtaříková 1996). Therefore, we have to look beyond medical care and health policy to determine why rising mortality among middle-aged working-class males was reversed.

Societal Stress

A reduction in stress does not seem to be the cause of decreasing mortality, either. Under late communism there were serious economic problems and the Czech Republic underwent the same collapse of communism and transition to a free-market economy as the other former socialist countries. But despite the sharing of the same stressful circumstances with its Soviet-bloc neighbors, life expectancy in the Czech Republic does not seem to have been harmed by a rise in mortality. The relatively rapid decline in deaths from nearly all causes for all age-groups after 1990 coincided with the rapid social transformation, economic insecurity, rise in unemployment, and stressful circumstances accompanying the postcommunist transition (Carlson and Rychtaříková 1996).

Some of the best research in this regard is that of Joseph Hraba and his associates (1996) who surveyed a random sample of Czech households in both 1990 and 1991 in relation to workplace and social network (family and friends) stressors. Although stress was reported, overall levels were not dramatically high—even though this was the early transition period to a free-market economy. There was also a lack of gender differences in that Czech men and women reported similar levels of exposure to stress and similar reactions to it. This pattern differs significantly from the United States where men are more stressed by the workplace and women by social network events. As Hraba et al. point out, gender role convergence in the workplace under socialism caused Czech women and men to be equally exposed in the labor market to the stress of economic reforms. Women also faced job insecurity, and the loss of their income was as much a financial problem for families as that of men. Gender roles in the workplace likely influenced the findings in this study as Hraba and his associates (1996:528) concluded that "there were no gender differences in exposure to stress, vulnerability to stress, in the effects of mastery and social support on distress symptoms, and there was no gender pattern of internal versus external distress symptoms." Consequently, these data do not show that men are more stressed than women, which makes it unlikely that men are more prone to premature deaths because of greater stress.

Health Lifestyles

The most probable origin of the increase in life expectancy in the Czech Republic lies in a phenomenon that bridges the political, social, and economic systems of communism and postcommunism. In previous chapters it was noted how lifestyle practices with unhealthy outcomes have been incorporated into the habitus of middle-aged working-class males. Excessive alcohol and cigarette consumption, fatty diets, and literally no leisure-time exercise, combined with the personal allocation of responsibility for health to the state, provided the structural context for lessened longevity. Given the reversal in rising mortality among the Czechs, can it be determined that lifestyles in the Czech Republic became healthier as well? The answer is yes, and evidence comes from several sources.

For example, in an important medical study of the decline in cardiovascular mortality of persons ages 25 to 64 in the Czech Republic between 1984 and 1993, Z. Škodová et al. (1997) found that favorable lifestyle changes had indeed occurred. Smoking among men had decreased and significant changes in the Czech diet had taken place, namely reductions in the consumption of meat (13%), milk and dairy products (26.8%), and butter (43.6%), and increases in the consumption of vegetable fats (16%), vegetables (8%), and tropical fruit (43.2%). Škodová and her colleagues (1997:374) credit these changes with having a positive impact on lowering the prevalence of high cholesterol in the population.

Other research supports the Škodová et al. findings concerning the decline in smoking for men and the decrease in the consumption of meat, dairy products, and fats (Institute of Health Information and Statistics of the Czech Republic 1995; Sekula, Babinska, and Petrova 1997). It has been observed elsewhere, for instance, that since 1989 there has been a substantial decline in levels of cholesterol and obesity consistent with national trends in food consumption and lower mortality from heart disease (Bobák et al. 1997). An important factor in this development is that the choice and accessibility of fruits and vegetables increased significantly after the fall of communism. In fact, the quality of food generally has improved dramatically and people have been better able to practice good nutrition. As for smoking, the Czechs used to have one of the highest male mortality rates in Europe from lung cancer caused by smoking; this situation, however, has improved markedly since the late 1980s (Kubik et al. 1995; Marel et al. 1996). The proportion of male smokers has declined nationally from 49.6% in 1985 to 43.9% in 1992. For females, the proportion of smokers has actually risen slightly from 27.4% in 1985 to 28.8% in 1992. Smoking still remains a major health problem but there are clear signs of downturn in male cigarette use consistent with a rise in longevity.

The most comprehensive study of Czech health lifestyles to date is a nationwide survey conducted by the Institute of Health Information and Statistics of the Czech Republic (1995) in 1993. With respect to diet, there were several expressions of positive food habits. For example, some 77.6% of the men and 90.6% of the women ate fruit daily in the summer, some 65.6% of the men and 77% of the women ate raw vegetables nearly every week in the winter, and a majority favored vegetable fats in cooking and in their diet. On the other hand, nearly half of the men and women consumed potato chips more than twice a week. Nevertheless, there appeared to be an awareness of dietary principles and a consideration of proper eating habits in their food consumption. Some 7.8% of the men in this study reported regular hard sports training, 26.9% engaged in recreational sports and exercise (jogging, heavy gardening), 35.3% in light activities (walking, bicycling), and 30% in sedentary activities (reading, watching television); of the women, 1.9% participated in hard sports training, 18% in recreational sports, 38.7% in light activities, and 41.4% were sedentary. These are much higher proportions of people engaging in physical activity than shown in previous studies for Russia and Hungary.

Some 40.5% of the men and 29.5% of the women were found to be current smokers in the survey. Compared to the 1992 figures discussed earlier, these data for 1993 suggest that male smoking has continued to fall and female smoking has continued to increase slightly. The greatest proportion of regular smokers among both men and women are in the 35–44 age-group. But again, we see decreasing levels of smoking consistent with declining rates of male mortality from cardiovascular diseases. Finally, in regard to alcohol consumption, some 93.8% of the men and 86.5% of the women drank, with 15.7% of the men and 1.8% of the women classified as heavy drinkers. Although a considerable proportion of the Czech population drinks, the style of drinking varies significantly from that in Russia and northwest Europe. While alcohol abuse is a significant social and health problem, the binge or episodic drinking that occurs in Russia is not as common among the Czechs. Czechs prefer beer (over 70% of all alcoholic beverages consumed) and typically drink it at mealtime with food.

This nationwide survey also showed important class differences. People at the upper end of the social scale were significantly more likely to be engaged in healthier lifestyle practices than people at the lower end. The key variable in this regard was education. Better-educated respondents, in comparison to those with less education, observed more healthy eating habits; they also smoked less and were more accepting of antismoking information. When it came to alcohol consumption, people with higher education, primarily males, were split into two extremes—frequent drinkers and abstainers—similar to the West. Other research confirms that Czechs with university and secondary levels of education practice the healthiest lifestyles (Bobák et al. 1997).

Overall, these data indicate that health lifestyles in the Czech Republic are not only healthier than those in Russia, Poland, and Hungary, but that levels of participation began to expand in the late 1980s and accelerated in the 1990s. It is not surprising then that the Czechs are the first to reverse their mortality pattern from a negative to a positive direction. Of all the former Soviet-bloc nations, the Czechs were the only ones to forge a largely industrial society early in the twentieth century. This fostered an educated population with a modern outlook. While communism suppressed initiative and required patients to be relatively passive recipients of health care, postcommunism has promoted greater individual responsibility for one's own health, lay self-care, and care by family members (Heitlinger 1993). The significance of health lifestyles in improving life expectancy in the Czech Republic goes well beyond the Czech experience to indicate the powerful role (either positive or negative) that lifestyles play in determining the health profile of individuals and large populations.

THE SLOVAK REPUBLIC

At the beginning of 1993 the Slovak people finally realized their desire for independence by establishing their own republic under its first president, Michael Kovac. A small nation, with a 1995 population of 5.4 million people, Slovakia has a developed agricultural system, industry, and natural resources. According to Kirschbaum (1995:273): "As a nation, the Slovaks are sufficiently homogeneous and educated to organize and run an efficient economy, to manage the environment, and to ensure social development that one expects of a modern society and economy." However, in the years since independence the economy has struggled and remains in the shadow of the Czech Republic. The Czechs have preferred to import German and Austrian goods, and new markets for Slovak exports have been difficult to find. Moreover, much of Slovakia's industry was oriented toward military production for which there is no longer high demand. Inflation has been around 20%, unemployment is relatively high at 15%, and the privatization of state enterprises has been slow. Consequently, Slovakia continues to face serious economic challenges in its transition to a free-market economy.

Male life expectancy remains one of the lowest in Europe but has improved somewhat since the communist period. Table 8.5 shows that in 1991 Slovak males lived an average of 66.7 years—the same as in 1970 (see table 8.1). However, by 1995 male longevity had improved to 68.5 years and appears to be consistently moving upward. For females, life expectancy increased only slightly from 75.4 years in 1990 to 76.3 years in 1995. Overall, the longevity trends in Slovakia, while on the positive side, are sluggish. The lowest male life expectancy occurs in the agricultural districts of southern Slovakia, which have a large Hungarian minority and a high percentage of men with the lowest educational status (Ginter 1997). A surprising paradox in Slovakia is that life expectancy is longest in the areas with the highest emissions of pollutants (Ginter, Tatara, and Sipekiová 1995).

Table 8.5

Life Expectancy in the Slovak Republic, 1990–1995

Year	Males	Females
1990	66.6	75.4
1991	66.7	75.2
1992	67.6	76.2
1993	68.3	76.7
1994	68.3	76.5
1995	68.5	76.3

SOURCE: Statistical Office of the Slovak Republic 1997.

Many physicians have gone into private practice and are paid either through contracts with health insurance companies or direct payments from patients; medical facilities, however, generally remain under state ownership because of a lack of funds to purchase them (Marrée and Groenewegen 1997). The largest health care insurer is the independent General Health Insurance Fund (GHIF) established in 1993, but additional private health insurance companies have been legally authorized since 1995. Insurance premiums are 13.7% of a worker's wages, with the employee paying 3.7% and the employer 10% of the assessment. Self-employed persons pay the full 13.7% of the amount assessed. As in the Czech Republic, the state pays the health insurance premiums for children, the elderly, and the unemployed. The central government also provides a budget for hospitals but most hospitals are struggling financially. In 1994, some 5.96% of the GDP was spent on health care.

While extensive data on health conditions in the Slovak Republic are lacking, current studies identify health lifestyles as the primary social determinant of life expectancy. Emil Ginter (1997), for example, has identified a wide disparity in male life expectancy within Slovakia. The difference in male longevity at birth is almost 6 years between the districts with the highest and the lowest life expectancy. The worst life expectancy is found among the Hungarian minority, people with low education, and those who work in agriculture, all of which, as noted, tend to be concentrated in the south. Slovaks, better-educated persons, and industrial workers have the highest longevity. Although the agricultural districts of southern Slovakia have drinking water contaminated with higher levels of nitrates than elsewhere in the republic, Ginter identifies the health lifestyles of the Hungarian minority as the principal culprit in the poor health of the region. "The life style of this minority," states Ginter (1997:135), "resembles the life style of Hungarians living in Hungary (i.e., a high consumption of tobacco, alcohol, salt, and pig meat)."

The most important single variable in determining life expectancy in Slovakia is education. Ginter points out that people with low education succumb much more easily to the pressures of totalitarian power and in the process become passive about their health. For Slovakia in particular and the former socialist countries in general, Ginter concludes that differences in life expectancy are a major result of poor health lifestyles. "One of the main reasons," states Ginter (1997:135), "for the short life expectancy in the former communist countries is unhealthy life style adopted by the population group with a low educational status; a high consumption of alcoholic beverages, especially hard drinks, a high consumption of cigarettes and unbalanced nutrition (i.e. a high consumption of animal fats, a low consumption of fruits and vegetables)." The slight improvement in the still relatively low Slovakian male life expectancy can be linked to a decline in tobacco sales and leveling off of mortality from lung cancer (Kubik et al. 1995), a decrease in alcohol consumption since 1990 (Szantova et al. 1997), and a small decline in cardiovascular mortality since 1991 (Báska and Straka 1995).

Chapter 9

Romania

In each of the former socialist countries discussed thus far, the long-term decline in life expectancy has shown either recent (Russia, Hungary, and Poland) or definite (Czech Republic and Slovakia) signs of improvement. This is not the case in Romania. Mortality is continuing to rise and male life expectancy to decline. In fact, longevity among Romanian males is lower in the mid-1990s than it was in the mid-1960s. The health crisis in Romania is clearly not over and this chapter explains why this is the case.

HEALTH AND SOCIAL CHANGE

Romania was an independent kingdom 100 years ago. But its modern origins go back to the Roman Empire's province of Dacia, which gives present-day Romanians more of a Latin than Slavic quality in appearance and language (Dogaru and Zahariade 1996). "Like the rest of the Balkans," states Flora Lewis (1987:468), "Romania was late in developing, cut off from the European mainstream by Turkish overlordship, with feudal habits and extremes of wealth and power." The society consisted of a small elite group of landowners who controlled a huge peasant class producing foodstuffs in an agrarian economic system. For over two centuries, the Romanian people had struggled to free themselves of Turkish rule through armed revolt and negotiation. By the mid-1800s, with the Ottoman Empire weakening, the Romanians were able to establish an

This chapter was written with the assistance of Daniela Vâlceanu, M.D., Institute of Health Services Management, Bucharest, Romania.

autonomous principality under nominal Turkish control. Despite a tradition of conflict with the Russians, Romania joined the side of Russia in a successful war against Turkey in 1877 and was rewarded with full independence under the provisions of the Treaty of Berlin in 1878.

The Kingdom of Romania

In 1881, Romania became a kingdom and its Prince Carol was crowned King Carol I. Under his rule, Romania became a viable national entity; some industries were developed, railroads constructed, modern banking and other financial services established, and a tiny middle class of largely Jewish merchants and factory owners emerged (Graham 1982). Concerned with the power politics exercised in the Balkans by the Austro-Hungarian and Russian Empires, Romania sought closer relationships with the West, especially France. Many scientific and technical terms had no equivalent in the old Romanian language and French was widely adopted. "French influence in late-nineteenth century Romania extended far beyond language; it was reflected in dress, in architecture (especially in the design of streets, buildings, and parks for Bucharest), in the arts—literature, painting, and music" (Graham 1982:10).

King Carol I died in 1916 and was succeeded by his nephew, King Ferdinand I. Romania stayed out of World War I until 1916, when it joined the Western and Russian allies against Austria-Hungary and Germany in the hope of acquiring new land. The war turned out to be a disaster initially. The Romanian army fared poorly, the Germans invaded and the Russians came to meet them in battle, but Bucharest fell and much of the country came under German occupation. When Russia was knocked out of the war by the 1917 Russian Revolution, Romania was forced to surrender. However, the defeat of Germany and Austria-Hungary in 1918 led Romania to renew the war by invading Hungary, which allowed them to acquire additional territory—including the province of Transylvania, which had been part of Romania in the middle ages, along with Bessarabia, Banat, and Bucovina. Romania literally doubled in size and population overnight. But, as E. Garrison Walters (1988:220) points out, the acquisition of new territory had a dark side: Large numbers of extremely hostile Hungarians and Germans were forcibly given the status of Romanian citizens and became disruptive elements in Romanian society in the interwar years.

In the 1920s and 1930s, Romania was perhaps the most backward country in Eastern Europe. Some 72% of the population was dependent upon agriculture for their livelihood, but there was only one tractor for every 2,500 farm workers (Walters 1988). Land reform in 1921 redistributed some 30% of the landholdings to peasants, but this measure failed to improve agricultural production because the small farms (each about 5 hectares) were unable to do more than barely support the families that owned them. Even after reform, as Walters explains, some 28% of the land was held by only four-tenths of 1% of the landowners. So the powerful landlords' interests remained generally intact, but much of their land was not cultivated and instead preserved as forests. "Overall," states Walters (1988:221), "agriculture, which should have been a strength of the Romanian economy, was even weaker than before [land reform]." Romania's industrial base, in contrast, was relatively strong largely because the country was one of Europe's leading oil producers. The export of other raw materials such as timber, metals, and minerals also generated income for the Romanian economy.

The social structure that emerged at this time was very similar to that of Hungary, with a small, wealthy, landowning nobility dominating politics and maintaining themselves at the top rung of the social ladder over several generations. Next were a less affluent and numerically small group of landed gentry owning medium-sized estates, followed by small middle and working classes, with the remaining population—about 77% of Romanian society—in the lowest stratum as peasant farmers (Graham 1982; Walters 1988). The peasants were extremely poor and produced little for the marketplace. They lived on a subsistence diet lacking in protein, and their overall level of health was not good. As for health care, a national health insurance system modeled after Bismarck's system in Germany was initiated prior to World War II. Only blue-collar workers, merchants, and employers and their families were covered. A premium based on income was paid in equal proportions by employers and employees; however, only some 5% of the population was covered by health insurance (WHO 1996).

In the aftermath of World War I, a communist party was formed and began agitating for power, only to be outlawed by the government in 1924. Numerous other political parties, representing a wide variety of interests, caused a turbulent political scene in the 1920s and 1930s. King Ferdinand's son, Carol II, a notorious playboy, had been forced to renounce his right to the throne in favor of his son Michael, but he maneuvered himself back into power and was crowned in 1930. In the meantime, an extremely violent fascist and anti-Semitic terrorist group known as the Iron Guard emerged. Allied with the Nazis, it became very powerful and caused considerable instability, including the murder of many people considered its enemies. Romania itself was increasingly dominated by Nazi Germany politically and economically. Dissatisfied with Romania's support for his policies, Adolf Hitler pressured King Carol II in 1940 to give Bessarabia and northern Bucovina to the Soviet Union in order to avoid a Soviet-Romanian confrontation. The Hungarians, in turn, seized Transylvania and the Bulgarians occupied southern Dobrudja. The intense negative reaction in Romania forced Carol to abdicate. His son Michael became king, but the government was controlled by a military dictatorship established by Marshal Ion Antonescu.

The new regime launched a reign of terror against its opponents. The Iron Guard turned against Antonescu only to be destroyed by the Romanian army with the assistance of the Germans. Antonescu brought Romania into World War II on the side of Germany and provided more manpower for the 1941 invasion of the Soviet Union than all other Axis allies combined. However, after the German defeat at Stalingrad in 1942, resulting in enormous casualties for the Romanians, it became increasingly clear that they were on the wrong side. A coup mounted by forces loyal to King Michael arrested Antonescu in 1944 and Romania declared war on Germany, placing its army under Soviet command. Soviet troops occupied the country and Romanian communists filled virtually all of the key government posts. Transylvania was returned to Romania, but the other lands taken by Russia and Bulgaria were lost. To the communists, the continuation of Romania as a monarchy was out of the question, and by 1947 King Michael had been forced to abdicate under the threat of civil war.

The Communist Period

Under the leadership of Gheorge Gheorgiu-Dej, Romania was transformed into a Stalinist-style socialist state. Private property was confiscated, police-state repression implemented, and a centrally controlled and nationalized economy established. The socioeconomic basis of capitalism was completely destroyed and a system of state farms and cooperatives organized for peasants. The previous social system was completely dismantled, with the old ruling elite eliminated as a dominant class. Under the communists, the proportion of peasants decreased from

77% in 1938 to 44% in 1972; about 42% of the population was urban and 58% rural (Graham 1982). Romania thus retained much of its agrarian character. However, the working class comprised some 26% of the population as industrial development continued, while the remaining 30% was divided between white-collar workers (especially government civil servants), technical specialists, the intelligentsia, managers of state enterprises, and a small *nomenklatura* of leading party officials at the top of society.

The collectivization of agriculture turned out to be a major undertaking that took 17 years (1950–67) to complete. The old landed aristocracy was easily removed by force through imprisonment or exile. But the peasants resisted collectivization, causing the process to move very slowly. Over 3 million peasant families were eventually removed from their small plots of land and placed on large collective farms owned by the state. For a predominantly rural society, the transformation of agricultural production from a private to a socialist system was a radical social change destroying centuries of tradition.

The Soviet Union had wanted Romania to remain primarily agricultural in order to stimulate trade by providing farm produce to the Soviet bloc and purchasing manufactured goods in return. However, the break between Stalin and Tito in Yugoslavia encouraged Gheorgiu-Dej to begin showing some independence from Moscow. On one hand Gheorgiu-Dej demonstrated loyalty to Moscow; on the other hand, he began distancing himself from Moscow's policies. After Stalin's death, he purged the Romanian Communist Party of opponents, moved to establish heavy industry so Romania could be self-sufficient, and sometimes refused to follow the Soviet Union's lead in foreign policy. These measures were highly popular with the Romanian people, who did not wish to be Soviet puppets. Furthermore, he negotiated the withdrawal of Soviet troops in 1957 and prohibited Warsaw Pact maneuvers on Romanian territory in 1962. According to Flora Lewis, Romania had a relationship with the Warsaw Pact that was similar to that of France with NATO. Romania was a difficult, prickly, and uncooperative ally, but an ally nevertheless. Lewis (1987:480) states:

> By 1964 the schism reached a point of openly declared policy. The Romanian party proclaimed that "there cannot be a father party and a son party, a superior party and a subordinate party, only a great family of Communist and worker parties with equal rights." It was called a Romanian declaration of independence, a claim to follow the party's "own

road to socialism," as the Yugoslav and Italian Communists had done before. But unlike the other quarrels between Communist leaders and Moscow, it advanced no real issue of ideology, no departures in the theory or practice of "building socialism" and brought no internal innovations.

Basically, what Gheorgiu-Dej's policies accomplished was to make himself extremely powerful within his own country and Romania somewhat independent internationally while remaining in the Soviet camp. Gheorgiu-Dej died in 1965 and was eventually succeeded by Nicolae Ceausescu, who came from a poor family and had little education. He had been a communist since his teenage years when he was recruited in jail while serving a sentence for theft. Ceausescu continued Romania on the same maverick course, developing friendly relations with communist China after its split from Moscow, improving relations with the West, ruthlessly repressing all internal dissent, and initiating extravagant development projects at the expense of living standards (Lewis 1987; Walters 1988). When Warsaw Pact countries invaded Czechoslovakia in 1968, Ceausescu refused to provide Romanian soldiers. Furthermore, he instigated a cult-like approach to rule, having himself depicted in the media, as Lewis (1987:481) observes, as "the supreme leader," "great thinker of the universe," "a lay God," and a "luminous beacon." He made his wife, Elena, his vice premier, and she also insisted on being treated as a supreme being. According to Gale Stokes (1993:158), Ceausescu's regime in the 1980s "became one of the world's most notorious dictatorships, and he himself as far removed from reality as any ruler in modern times."

Ceausescu embarked upon highly ambitious building programs, using money that could have been spent upon improving Romania's deteriorating living conditions. He had part of old Bucharest razed and some of its most historic houses destroyed in order to build large and impressive government buildings and wide avenues. Today, most of these buildings remain unfinished, with gutted interiors and broken windows. The Romanian government has neither the money to finish them, nor a use for them if completed. In the meantime, gasoline, electricity, central heating, and food were in short supply. Electric heaters were banned and refrigerators had to be unplugged in the winter. Television was broadcast only two hours nightly, often consisting of one hour of news about Ceausescu and his family and a second hour of Ceausescu addressing the nation. In order to repay loans from the West, Ceausescu sold much of Romania's farm produce abroad and introduced food rationing in 1981. In 1982, Ceausescu created a

Rational Nourishment Commission to reduce the country's caloric intake through a program of "rational eating," which many Romanians felt was more about "rationing" than "eating." As Lewis (1987:482) comments:

> When food shortages became acute, Ceausescu announced that 30% of illness throughout the country was due to gluttony. He prescribed a "scientific diet" for health purposes. It permitted, per month, 10 eggs, ¼ pound of butter, 2.2 pounds of cooking oil and 2.2 pounds of meat—though he did not say how these items were to be found in the empty markets.

According to Stokes (1993:158), for the remainder "of the 1980s the food situation for ordinary Romanians deteriorated so dramatically that by the end of the decade simply getting any kind of food required substantial effort for every family." Consequently, the concept of dieting in Romania has been discredited and, even today, is not used in public health campaigns. To a people with relatively recent memories of coping with semi-starvation, the notion of dieting in order to be healthy is an anathema.

Under these circumstances it would appear likely that Romania's health care delivery system lacked adequate financial support. And this was indeed the case. Beginning in 1949, Romania converted to a Soviet-style health care system. This meant a hierarchical, centralized system utilizing dispensaries as the entry point to patient services. Private care was abolished, physicians and other health care workers became state employees, and the state assumed ownership of all facilities. There was free, universal coverage with the costs paid by the central government. The best physicians, hospitals, and clinics were reserved for Ceausescu, his family, and the elite of the Communist Party. Moreover, starting in 1983, as Ceausescu was stripping his country of resources to pay foreign debts, out-of-pocket payments for some health services were required of patients—even though all treatment was provided in state-owned facilities. Within the system, efforts were made to compensate for the lack of material quality by increasing the number of low-paid health care workers. Gifts or payments by patients in the form of gratuities insured more personalized attention and supplemented the low incomes of providers.

The overall quality of care was poor because of underfunding, inadequate equipment and facilities, inefficiency, and a lack of individual initiative by health administrators and providers (WHO 1996). For example, between 1985 and 1989 government expenditures on health averaged 2.2% of the GDP, which is a lower percentage than that in the other

Central and Eastern European countries (Vâlceanu 1992). The Ministry of Health was also responsible for some nonmedical institutions, such as orphanages and day nurseries for working mothers, so expenditures on medical services were actually even lower than that. As a "nonproductive" sector of the economy, requiring money rather than generating it, health care was accorded a low priority in the nation's budget distribution.

As seen in table 9.1, life expectancy in Romania in 1961 was 64.2 years for males and 67.7 years for females. Male life expectancy reached 66.4 years in 1964–67, dropped slightly to 66.3 years in 1970–72, and climbed to a high of 67.4 years in 1976–78. At this point, the mid- to late 1970s, Romanian male longevity began a consistent decline and stood at 66.3 years in 1986–88. Female life expectancy has fared better, rising from 67.7 years in 1961 to 72.3 in 1986–88. While the overall increase for women is not impressive in relation to the West, it nevertheless is on the plus of longevity and outperforms male life expectancy by nearly 6 years between the early 1960s and the end of communist rule in 1989. As in the other former socialist countries, the most important contribution to the deterioration of life expectancy in Romania is the increase in mortality among adult males (Muresan 1996).

Table 9.1

Life Expectancy in Romania, 1961–1996

Year	Males	Female
1961	64.2	67.7
1964–67	66.4	70.5
1970–72	66.3	70.9
1972–74	66.8	71.3
1974–76	67.4	72.0
1976–78	67.4	72.2
1978–80	66.7	71.8
1980–82	66.7	72.2
1982–84	67.0	72.6
1984–86	66.8	72.8
1986–88	66.3	72.3
1988–90	66.6	72.7
1990–92	66.6	73.2
1992–94	65.9	73.3
1996	65.5	73.6

SOURCE: Romanian Ministry of Health.

Public criticism of conditions and protest in Romania were muted because of the strength and efficiency of the secret police. Intense state repression made it difficult for opposition to arise and, when protests and riots did occur, police repression was swift, violent, and effective; the leaders would disappear and the events would go unreported in the media (Stokes 1993). Gorbachev's policies of *glasnost* and *perestroika* in the Soviet Union were rejected by Ceausescu, who maintained that each socialist country had the right to decide on its own course of development. In November of 1989, even though the Berlin Wall had fallen, neighboring Bulgaria had replaced its communist leader, and huge street demonstrations were taking place in Prague, Romania appeared secure for the communists. Stokes (1993) indicates that it seemed unlikely the regime would be swept out of power by the same type of unrest occurring elsewhere in Eastern Europe. But Ceausescu's power was a facade, and when it was challenged, his government quickly and surprisingly disintegrated.

The collapse began in Timisoara in southwest Romania near the Serbian border, when an outspoken priest, László Tökés of the Hungarian Reformed Church, was ordered to leave. Tökés insisted that only his congregation could dismiss him and crowds gathered to protect him when the police were sent to forcibly remove him. On 17 December 1989 the army entered Timisoara but did little until Ceausescu ordered them to attack the demonstrators that night. A massacre ensued in which at least 97 people were killed (Stokes 1993). Ceausescu then left the country for a two-day state visit to Iran. In the meantime, a workers' strike paralyzed Timisoara, the local government was ousted by angry crowds, and the army withdrew, no longer willing to shoot Romanians. Demonstrations and strikes spread to other cities. Ceausescu returned and ordered a televised mass meeting of loyal supporters in the center of Bucharest on 21 December. This move backfired when thousands of people began shouting in front of a nationwide audience, calling him a dictator. He had treated so many people so badly for so long that widespread support was absent. Fighting broke out between the army and the secret police. The next day, 22 December, Ceausescu again tried to speak to the crowd but fled by helicopter when demonstrators became unruly. He and his wife were captured shortly thereafter and executed by a firing squad on 25 December after a one-day trial. The army and the plotters associated with them did not take any chances on his returning to power.

Postcommunist Romania

Following the fall of Ceausescu, Ion Iliescu, a middle-range Communist Party official, formed a new postcommunist government as president. Since dissident groups did not exist, the army, secret police, and former communist bureaucrats agreed to support Iliescu. The economic situation, however, did not improve markedly in the first few years after communism. The government was reluctant to initiate reforms that might prove unpopular. A few people, namely a small group of well-placed former communist officials, became wealthy. Most people, however, fared poorly. Over half of Romania's 1995 population of 23.5 million people lived below the official poverty line of $160 monthly and many households spent as much as 70% of their income on food, thereby suggesting that Romania's evolving postcommunist class structure contains a relatively high proportion (50% or more) of socially and economically disadvantaged persons. Privatization was the slowest in the former Soviet bloc.

Change came in 1996 when Emil Constantinescu was elected president and Victor Carbea became prime minister. The new government set about bringing reform by raising interest rates, cutting subsidies to industrial companies (an expense that had consumed as much as 10% of the national budget), and reducing government spending. Privatization was accelerated as the share of the private sector increased from 52% in 1996 to 66% in 1997. The sales of several large state enterprises to private interests were part of this increase. Unemployment rates dropped from 12.9% in 1994 to 6.8% in 1997, one of the lowest in Europe. The GDP improved from a decrease of 15% in 1994 to an increase of 4.1% in 1996. Consequently, Romania's economic prospects appear more positive in the late 1990s.

As for life expectancy, the pattern of male longevity continued its decline in the early 1990s and it is too early to assess whether improved economic conditions will promote longer lives for Romanian men by the end of the decade. Table 9.1 shows that male life expectancy was frozen at 66.6 years in the early 1990s, but fell to 65.9 years in 1992–94 and to 65.5 years in 1996. Table 9.1 also shows that Romanian males lived longer on average in 1964–67 (66.4 years) than they did in 1996 (65.5 years). This situation represents an obvious tragedy for males. For females, life expectancy reached 73.6 years in 1996 as women continued to see a slow but steady increase since 1961.

Table 9.2 shows the major causes of mortality for both sexes in Romania between 1960 and 1995. In 1960, the death rate from all causes

Table 9.2

Selected Major Causes of Death per 100,000 Persons, Romania, 1960–95

Cause	1960	1965	1975	1985	1989	1990	1991	1992	1993	1994	1995
All causes	873.3	858.7	929.8	1085.5	1068.2	1064.7	1085.9	1159.9	1157.2	1157.2	1197.8
Tuberculosis	35.1	24.0	6.7	4.2	5.6	6.9	7.3	8.6	10.2	10.5	11.3
Cancer	108.9	123.0	129.3	136.7	141.6	142.1	144.7	153.0	158.9	162.2	165.5
Disease of the circulatory system	363.8	395.0	478.2	630.6	617.6	627.0	658.2	707.8	712.3	709.9	736.1
Diseases of the respiratory system	118.5	135.9	148.6	127.1	105.7	97.3	91.3	94.0	79.7	80.6	75.8
Diseases of the digestive system	48.9	40.0	36.6	52.6	53.5	50.3	51.8	57.9	62.5	65.6	68.2
Accidents	43.7	52.6	61.6	67.8	74.7	76.5	72.8	74.3	73.8	76.1	78.6

SOURCE: Romanian Ministry of Health.

was 873.3 per 100,000 population and increased to 1,197.8 by 1995. Much of this rise was caused by deaths from diseases of the circulatory system, which increased from 363.8 per 100,000 persons in 1960 to 736.1 in 1995. Although there is a possibility that heart disease mortality may have been overdiagnosed under communist rule, 1990s data appear reasonably accurate. The general pattern is therefore clear: Cardiovascular problems are the leading cause of death in Romania and have continued to increase in occurrence since the 1960s. Table 9.2 also shows that deaths caused by cancer increased from 108.9 per 100,000 people in 1960 to 165.5 in 1995; by diseases of the digestive system from 48.9 to 68.2; and by accidents from 43.7 to 78.6. Tuberculosis mortality, which had declined from 35.1 per 100,000 in 1960 to 4.2 in 1985, began increasing again and stood at 11.3 deaths per 100,000 in 1995. However, under Ceausescu, there were not supposed to be any deaths from diseases related to social causes, like tuberculosis, in Romania's "perfect society." So the extent to which tuberculosis actually declined prior to the 1990s is questionable, but its increase after 1989 appears certain. Table 9.2 shows that it is only in diseases of the respiratory system that a decrease was registered, with the death rate dropping from 118.5 per 100,000 in 1960 to 75.8 in 1995. The overall mortality pattern for Romania is obviously negative and features a steady increase in all major causes of death, except respiratory diseases. Mortality rates from circulatory diseases literally doubled between 1960 and 1995.

THE SOCIAL DETERMINANTS OF LIFE EXPECTANCY

Given Romania's relatively poor health profile and generally substandard living conditions, it is not difficult to make a case for the importance of social factors in causing premature mortality among males. Biomedical factors like poor-quality medical care and the spread of infectious diseases—as seen in table 9.2 in the case of tuberculosis—may be important as well. But life expectancy for Romanian women has consistently risen while that for men was falling, so medical care alone does not seem a likely cause of early deaths for the population generally, unless, in some way, women receive better care than men, for which there is no evidence. Furthermore, any increase in infectious diseases would have affected women as well as men. And since mortality from respiratory diseases, which includes deaths from pneumonia and influenza, has consistently declined since 1960, a strong case for infectious diseases as a principal cause of rising mortality is seriously undermined. Consequently, I turn to the social determinants of policy, societal stress, and health lifestyles as the likely causal factors in the downturn in male life expectancy, and again argue that lifestyles are the ultimate determining factor.

Policy

Health policy in Romania has not been effective to date in curtailing the premature mortality of middle-aged males. The solution during the Ceausescu era, as noted, was to increase the number of health care workers to make up for shortages in funds, supplies, and medical equipment. This obviously did not work. In the aftermath of communism's collapse, the former Soviet-style health care system was maintained and continued to be financed by the central government. Health expenditures were only 2.9% of the GDP in 1990 and, as recently as 1996, have declined to 2.5%. In 1997, health expenditures were projected to rise to 3.4% of the GDP, but this is still a low percentage. Thus, the health system has continued to be seriously underfinanced in the postcommunist period. Budgets are provided to districts on a per capita basis, which means that the poorest parts of the country in the east and south receive the lowest budgets since they have less population; urban areas receive 87% of the total allocation, so a geographical inequity exists as well (Vâlceanu 1992).

Romanian citizens were entitled to free care in state-owned facilities; they paid 50% of the cost of prescribed drugs and gave co-payments for dental care, induced abortions, and hospital admissions without referrals from a physician. All hospitalization was provided in government-owned hospitals, but outpatient care was available in both private and public clinics. Patients paid 100% of their expenses in the private sector, which remains quite small (WHO 1996). Most of the state's medical budget (69%) went to fund the operation of hospitals and polyclinics, with a relatively small amount left over for primary care and health education (Vâlceanu 1992). The salaries of physicians continued to be supplemented by the payment of gratuities from patients.

However, a far-reaching change in the financing of health care that will transform the current system was passed by Romania's parliament in 1997. This was the passage of a measure authorizing the implementation of a national health insurance program. Beginning in 1998, all employees will pay 5% of their total earnings for compulsory health insurance to an insurance company, Casa de Asigurari pentru Sanatate. Employers also contribute an amount equal to 5% of their employees' wages. Retired persons will pay 4% of their income, while the unemployed and disabled will be covered by the state. The company, on its part, will purchase health care services from the state. Private care was not covered as this book went to press. Patients covered under the health insurance program will be able to choose the primary care doctor or hospital they go to for treatment, so, theoretically, the better physicians and hospitals should prosper while the poor ones should have to shut down. For the first time, free-market competition will be introduced into Romania's health care delivery system, which will hopefully result in improved services. The new system will begin its full operation in 1999 when the insurance company will have accumulated enough funds to pay providers.

The national health insurance law is the first reform measure in health care since the beginning of communist rule in 1947. It was long overdue because of the poor state of the health care system. Other reforms are underway to improve primary care, expand health education programs, increase health planning at local levels, and extend national health insurance to private practitioners and hospitals. Taxes on alcohol and tobacco have been raised in an attempt to reduce their use. However, the health care system remains overcentralized and under-funded to date. Whether or not the national health insurance plan will be able to funnel significantly more money into the health system is not known at present—although expectations are that it will. There are also serious problems of equity. The quality of care remains higher in urban areas; also, patients with higher incomes, who can afford "under-the-table" payments, have received preferential treatment from doctors in the past, making it harder for low- and medium-income patients to receive quality care (Vâlceanu 1992). The extent to which the practice of gratuities will continue under national health insurance is not known, although the income of competent doctors should rise as they attract more patients with insurance.

Health policy in Romania is now oriented toward reform. Public health goals, however, need to be further clarified based upon accurate data about health conditions. In the meantime, can it be claimed that rising mortality for Romanian males has been caused by the country's past health policies? The answer is no. The critical mortality characteristics of male sex, middle age, manual work, and heart disease do not originate in policy decisions that affect men and women alike. Romania's health policy has failed to cope with the rise of chronic disease but, while the relatively low quality of services undoubtedly produced cases of avoidable mortality, there is no evidence that policy is the primary cause of the downturn in male life expectancy. Heart disease is not caused by poor medical care.

Societal Stress

There is a complete absence of research in Romania on the health effects of stress. While a case for stressful societal conditions can be made, it is not at all clear that stress is killing middle-aged males prematurely in any direct manner. For example, research on the effects of stress from the December 1989 uprising in the city of Cluj against Ceausescu's forces did not find a higher incidence of heart attacks or increased hospital admissions for cardiovascular complaints (Dumitrascu, Hopulele, and Baban 1993). The transition to a free-market economy has most likely promoted a sense of loss regarding the social security of communism (guaranteed jobs, pensions, and health care, along with price controls on rent and food), an unstable environment, feelings of uncertainty, loss of self-esteem, difficulty in handling personal freedom, and an inability to generate alternatives to problems and coping with them. But whether these stressors are responsible for the consistent decline in male (but not female) longevity is not known. Such stresses may, in fact, be lessening as the economy improves and unemployment declines. A problem with the stress explanation for Romania is that its effects are difficult to isolate from the intervening contributions of lacking social support, bad living conditions, poor-quality medical care, and unhealthy lifestyles. As stated in earlier chapters, the role of societal-level stress may have been greatest in promoting excessive alcohol and cigarette consumption, along with other unhealthy lifestyle practices. However, this conclusion needs to be confirmed by research findings and, to date, such research has not been conducted in Romania.

Health Lifestyles

There is also a lack of data on health lifestyles in Romania, but some information exists. Some background information is provided by a 1995 nationwide survey of self-rated health statuses (Mihăilă, Enăchescu, and Bădulescu 1996). Urban residents at the top of the social scale with good jobs and education ranked their health the best; however, a comparison of Romanian scores with results from Switzerland, the United States, Sweden, and Great Britain showed that the Romanians realistically rank their health status much lower than respondents in these Western countries.

It is clear that the greatest contribution to rising mortality does not come from infants, children, adolescents and 20- to 34-year-old adult males, the elderly, or females; rather, it comes from the high percentage of deaths among 35- to 59-year-old males (Muresan 1996). It would therefore be expected that this particular age and gender group would have the highest levels of alcohol and cigarette consumption. Although little data are available, surveys conducted by the Central Statistical Office of the Ministry of Health (Centrul de Calcul si Statistica Sanitara 1992) indicate that 30- to 59-year-old males have a higher proportion of drinkers (83.1%) than younger (76.7%) or older males (63.4%), or women generally (46.9%). Beer is the preferred alcoholic beverage, followed by wine and hard liquor. When it comes to smoking, 20- to 29-year-old males have a slightly higher proportion of smokers (54.9%), but the 30- to 59-year-old males are close behind (52%). Among 60-and-over males, some 29.7% smoke. The total percentage of women smokers is low (13.3%).

Clearly, alcohol consumption and smoking are highest among middle-aged males. A firsthand account of the heavy drinking that takes place among some middle-aged male manual workers is provided by Robert Kaplan (1993), who traveled throughout Romania in the early 1990s. On a boat trip to the Danube delta on the Black Sea, Kaplan (1993:109–11) found that:

> almost all the men on this boat (and the men far outnumbered the women) were drunk and getting drunker, in a very unpleasant way. After the bar ran out of *tuica* [plum brandy], bottles were pulled out of burlap sacks. Some of these bottles contained homemade brandy; others, medical alcohol. As the crowd thinned out at halts along the way, I realized that the heaviest drinkers were staying aboard and congregating in the cabin, where bad weather on deck compelled me to go, too.
>
> The air in the cabin was an invisible wall that slammed me in the face. With the windows sealed shut, most of the free oxygen had been sucked out of the air, its place taken by carbon dioxide, vapors of brandy, and perspiration, and the vilest of tobacco fumes. A forest of empty bottles spread across the tables. . . . I closed my eyes and pretended to fall asleep. The drinking went on.
>
> Another of Ceausescu's legacies was this underclass straight out of George Orwell's *1984*: badly urbanized peasants who, according to a local proverb, were "neither horse nor donkey," uprooted from villages where

their ancestors had lived for decades or centuries—away from every tradition they ever had—and moved to factory dormitories where everything was in short supply except alcohol and regime propaganda.

Along with excessive drinking which remains a serious health problem for males, especially low-skilled, manual workers, smoking is also common among these men. A problem in curtailing smoking in Romania is that it is associated with status, especially if the cigarettes are of good quality and foreign. "Kent" cigarettes are the most popular and have been so for years. Sometimes they were used to barter for goods and services—including personalized medical care—when money was in short supply under Ceausescu. Although overall levels of smoking in Romania are not as high as in Poland and Hungary, more than half of all young and middle-aged adult Romanian males smoke, and it is among the middle-aged that smoking has its greatest and most adverse impact on health.

Data are also lacking on diet and exercise, although some dietary research shows that the consumption of cereal, potatoes, and meat declined between 1989 and 1992 and the intake of fats, sugar, and dairy products increased (Sekula, Babinska, and Petrova 1997). Throughout this period, the proportion of animal protein consumed was low and that of saturated fat very high. This diet has surely contributed to the continuing increased occurrence of heart disease. On practically every measure, the general Romanian diet has been poor for some years and is a major factor in the poor health of the population.

While less information on health lifestyles is available for Romania than for the other countries discussed thus far, it is obvious that the overall standard of living was low and it was perhaps impossible for most people to have a healthy lifestyle. The group most affected are, again, middle-aged working-class males. Therefore, the same general pattern of life expectancy common to the other former Soviet-bloc countries is repeated. While policy and stress are likely contributing factors, available data suggest that unhealthy lifestyle practices are the ultimate cause of the downturn in male longevity and that a general improvement in living standards and health-related behavior is needed to reverse this situation.

Chapter 10

Bulgaria

From the mid-1960s to the late 1990s, male life expectancy in Bulgaria has been slowly but continuously turning downward in a yet unbroken decline. Longevity for women, in contrast, has steadily increased during the same period. What is it about the health situation of Bulgarian males that has been cutting off their life expectancy for approximately 30 years? This chapter examines this question in a search for the answer.

HEALTH AND SOCIAL CHANGE

Bulgaria, with a 1994 population of 8.4 million people, is the southernmost Eastern European country and shares borders with Romania, Serbia, Macedonia, Greece, and Turkey. The original Bulgarian state was founded in 681 and was among the most powerful and advanced kingdoms of Europe in the early Middle Ages (Kaplan 1993). A predominantly Slavic nation, Bulgaria experienced cycles of regional power and decline before having its independence extinguished by the Turks in a series of battles fought between 1366 and 1396. The country was ruled by various Turkish overlords for nearly 500 years and cut off from the rest of Europe. Its population was generally relegated to the role of peasant farmers, and the arable land devoted to agriculture. As Robert Kaplan (1993:205) explains:

This chapter was written with the assistance of Nevyana Feschieva, M.D., Ph.D., Head, Department of Social Medicine and Biostatistics, Medical University, Varna, Bulgaria.

But unlike other countries whose empire peaked and gradually faded into oblivion, Bulgaria was then cut down in the prime of nationhood by a series of invasions that culminated in a 500-year-long Ottoman Turkish occupation. Because Bulgaria was used by the Turks as their principal military base for further expansion in Europe, Turkish rule was bloodier and more overbearing in Bulgaria than anywhere else. Whole populations were expelled from urban centers; forced labor was prescribed for conquered peasants, and the relatively advanced feudal system was replaced by a more primitive one. Along with Serbia, Bulgaria was the first Balkan nation to be conquered by the Turks, but it was the very last one to be liberated. "From 1393 until 1877 Bulgaria may truthfully be said to have had no history," writes [Nevill] Forbes.

Bulgarians had traditionally been difficult to rule, and throughout the Ottoman Empire's period of occupation there were uprisings and resistance. Growing discontent and feelings of nationalism fueled a major revolt in 1876, which the Turks once more ruthlessly suppressed. The plight of the Bulgarians encouraged Russia to go to war against Turkey in 1877 and the subsequent victory liberated Bulgaria and earned the lasting gratitude of the Bulgarian people. Even though Bulgaria was on the opposite side of Russia in both world wars, Bulgarians share a similar language and religion (Eastern Orthodox Church) with Russia, and Bulgaria ranked among the most loyal allies of the Soviet Union. Today, when Bulgarians refer to the liberation, they do not mean the end of communism but the independence from Turkey which restored their nationhood. The 1878 Treaty of Berlin, however, which formalized Bulgaria's independence, was bittersweet. A considerable portion of Bulgaria's historic territory was lost, including the emotionally charged cessation of the province of Macedonia which eventually became part of the former Yugoslavia.

The Precommunist Period

One hundred years ago Bulgaria was a constitutional monarchy ruled by a German, King Ferdinand I. The early years of the twentieth century were turbulent, both with respect to the country's internal politics and the involvement of Bulgaria in a successful war against Turkey (1912) and a major defeat at the hands of Greece and Serbia (1913). Hoping to regain Macedonia, Bulgaria entered World War I on the side of Germany and Austria-Hungary in 1916 and invaded Serbia. At first the war went well, but Bulgaria emerged on the losing side in 1918. King Ferdinand I was forced to abdicate in favor of his son Boris III and all territorial gains from the war were reversed.

The war itself caused deep divisions in Bulgarian society as the population generally desired the return of Macedonia but not warfare against other Slavs, namely Russia and Serbia. Bulgarian society between the two world wars should have been stable because of the relatively egalitarian class system, but it was not (Lewis 1987; Walters 1988). There was no native nobility as a Bulgarian elite class was not allowed to develop under the Turks. Land reform had not been difficult because the former large landowners had been Turks who were stripped of their property after independence. E. Garrison Walters (1988) points out that interwar Bulgaria was a thoroughly peasant society, with some 75% of the population dependent upon agriculture for their livelihood; there was little industry and little in the way of a middle class. Manufacturing consisted largely of textiles and handicrafts. "To the extent there were social classes in Bulgaria," states Walters (1988:251), "it was essentially a consequence of the difference between rich and poor peasants." Walters points out that even the small urban population was closely tied to a peasant lifestyle and that the society was as homogenous as its economy. Bulgaria, in Walters's (1988:51) view, "was a land of peasant proprietors." According to Flora Lewis (1987:495):

> The land reform had produced an agriculture based on small and medium holdings, with 98% of the farmers owning their own land. They lived on bread, potatoes, cheese, yogurt, and peppers, and only one village in nine had electricity on the eve of World War II. But they were diligent and industrious, open to improved techniques when those were available, and despite their poverty they had a sense of participation in the society. The achievement of independence in the nineteenth century had swept away the Turkish feudalism, so that the political, bureaucratic, and military elites were recruited from the peasants and artisans. The educational system was open and more widespread than in other countries in the area. The literacy rate was the highest in the Balkans. . . . [The Bulgarians] appreciated order, sobriety, practicality, innovation.

As for life expectancy, the Bulgarians were not especially long-lived. As seen in table 10.1, life expectancy for Bulgarian males rose from 44.3 years in 1921–25 to 51 years in 1935–39 and that for females from 45 years to 52.6 years during the same period. By way of comparison, in 1939 French males had a life expectancy of 56.5 years and French females of 62.6 years; American males lived 62.1 years and American females 65.4 years that same year. Consequently, in the late 1930s French men outlived their Bulgarian counterparts by 5.5 years and American men had a longevity advantage of 11 years. French women outlived Bulgarian women by an average of 6 years and American women by over 13 years.

Table 10.1

Life Expectancy in Bulgaria, 1921–1995

Year	Males	Females
1921–25	44.3	45.0
1927–34	47.6	49.1
1935–39	51.0	52.6
1956-57	64.2	67.6
1960–63	67.8	71.3
1965–67	68.8	72.7
1974–76	68.7	73.9
1978–80	68.3	73.5
1984–86	68.2	74.4
1989–91	68.0	74.7
1992	67.6	74.4
1991–93	67.7	74.7
1993–95	67.1	74.8

SOURCE: Bulgarian National Center of Health Informatics 1995.

Unfortunately, Bulgaria was not able to devote more resources toward improving health and life expectancy during the interwar period. An adequate health care system existed in the cities, but many peasants lacked convenient access to professional health care and utilized the services of traditional healers in their villages. The greatest problem facing the country was political conflict. As Walters (1988:253) explains, some people always seem to find reasons for strife, and the Bulgarians were no exception. Communists and other left-wing organizations, right-wing groups, Macedonian revolutionaries, urban-rural disputes over government decisions, and problems with the Turkish minority who constituted about 11% of the population—all were troublesome. In 1932 army officers launched a coup against the government and instigated a right-wing reign of terror. The communists responded with a badly prepared and poorly executed counterrevolution that was crushed. King Boris III, in turn, initiated his own coup in 1935 which established a royal dictatorship. He was sympathetic to Nazi Germany but resisted full collaboration and did not allow the deportation of Bulgaria's Jews to Nazi concentration camps; moreover, he declared war only on the Western allies in 1943, not the Soviet Union (Lewis 1987). Bulgaria's principal wartime activity was the occupation of Macedonia; otherwise, there was little fighting and minimal destruction in the country.

Following Boris's death by heart attack in 1943 after a difficult meeting with Hitler, Bulgaria was briefly ruled by a regency council who realized that the country was again on the wrong side in a world war and desperately tried to arrange an armistice. But the Soviet Union declared war on Bulgaria instead, and its armies swept through the country, aided by Bulgarian communist paramilitary units who insured relatively unimpeded progress. Under Soviet military occupation, the communists took power, abolished the monarchy, ousted anticommunist leaders, and executed opponents of the new regime and Nazi supporters. After that, as Lewis (1987:498) explains, there were no more Bulgarian politics. Debate was over and the country became a socialist republic in 1947. Kaplan (1993:207–8) adds:

> In terms of military occupation and loss of land, Soviet domination cost the Bulgarians little. Because their country was not contiguous to the Soviet Union, the Soviets had no territorial claims to make—unlike in the cases of Romania, Hungary, Czechoslovakia, and Poland, whom the Soviets forced to give up territory as the Soviet border moved westward after World War II. Located farthest away from the line of confrontation between East and West in Central Europe, Bulgaria was also the least strategically important of all the Warsaw Pact states. Thus, when local Communists consolidated control under the leadership of the Moscow-trained [Georgi] Dimitrov in December 1947, the Soviet army withdrew from Bulgaria, never to return except for yearly maneuvers. Bulgarians bristled at the claim they were "vassals" of the Soviets, pointing out that while Hungary (which through the 1970s and 1980s enjoyed a high reputation in the West) was hosting 60,000 Soviet soldiers on its soil, Bulgaria had no Soviet soldiers.
>
> Besides no troops, no loss of territory, and positive historical memories, the Russians offered Bulgaria a heady psychological brew: guaranteed protection against Turkey; and numerous opportunities to deal with that hated former colonial master from a position of strength, not weakness. As a Bulgarian diplomat once told me: "It is the bear that protects us from the barking dog."

The Communist Period

Bulgaria began its existence as a communist state with internal purges and "show trials" of party members in the Stalinist style. Eventually, beginning in 1954, Todor Zhivkov, the son of a poor peasant family, came to power through astute political maneuvering within the communist hierarchy. Under Zhivkov, who maintained his leadership position for 35 years until 1989, Bulgaria evolved as a dependable ally of the Soviet Union in return for economic support. Because of its relatively backward agrarian economy, Bulgaria escaped much of the heavy industrialization that was emphasized by the Soviets elsewhere in Eastern Europe. Faithfully following the Soviet model, Bulgaria collectivized its agriculture to the point that by 1958 over 90% of its arable land was under cultivation by state farms. Bulgaria became a major source of food for the former Soviet bloc and generally provided its own people with a varied and relatively healthy diet (Lewis 1987). Industrialization did occur, however, and the production of machine tools, metallurgy, and chemicals, along with food, beverage, and tobacco processing, was developed. Yet Bulgaria's major products remained foodstuffs; over half of its exports went to the Soviet Union and another 25% to Eastern Europe. Economic development was steady and supported by loans from the Soviets, thereby allowing Bulgaria to escape massive debts to the West during the communist era. But Bulgaria owed huge debts to the Soviet Union and was so closely tied to the Soviet economy that its own economic system began to falter when the Soviet version turned downward. The decreased ability of the Soviets to purchase Bulgarian goods had a significant and adverse impact on Bulgaria's economy. Even today, the loss of the market in the former Soviet Union has a huge negative impact on Bulgaria's trade.

In the meantime, Bulgaria's society was transformed into a Soviet-style social system with the typical communist class structure consisting of the *nomenklatura*, managers of state enterprises, the intelligentsia, technical specialists and white-collar workers, the industrial working class, and peasants. The largest social stratum was the working class, as Bulgaria's urban population grew to over 60% under the communists. The health care delivery system was based on the Soviet Union's Semashko model with a hierarchical system of hospitals and polyclinics, free health care, state ownership of facilities and employment of doctors and other health care workers, centralized management and planning, and a focus on primary care and prevention. Shortcomings were similar to those in the other former socialist countries, namely rigid planning, low salaries and low professional satisfaction for physicians, gratuities for more personal care, oversupply of health care workers in hospitals and polyclinics, unrealistic objectives, ineffective health promotion activities, and shortages of qualified doctors in rural areas (Borissov and Rathwell 1996). Most rural health care was performed by physician assistants, rather than physicians, and rural care was not generally considered adequate for the needs of the population (Minev, Dermendjieva, and Mileva 1990). The percentage of the GDP spent on health in 1988, however, was 4.2, which was low in relation to the West but among the highest levels of health expenditures in the former Soviet bloc at that time. Nevertheless, not enough of the GDP was spent on health during the communist period; among several problems were the lack of construction of new health care facilities, and a failure to improve conditions within the existing facilities (Minev et al. 1990).

Table 10.1 shows that life expectancy for Bulgarian males in 1956–57 was 64.2 years and for females 67.6 years. This was a considerable improvement since the late 1930s and suggests that Soviet-style health care, with its emphasis on curtailing infectious diseases and reducing infant mortality, was effective in the late 1940s and 1950s. By 1965–67, male longevity peaked at 68.8 years and thereafter entered a steady but gradual decline that reached 68 years (a loss of 0.8 years) at the end of the communist era (1989–91). While this decrease is considerably less than that in the Soviet Union, it is still a loss (actually more of a stagnation), and compares very unfavorably with the life expectancy of French males during the same period. In 1967 the life expectancy of French men was a year less (67.8 years) than that of Bulgarian men (68.8 years), but while Bulgarian male longevity fell 0.8 years, that of French males increased by 5.1 years to 72.9 years by 1991. Clearly, "something" had happened that arrested the life expectancy of Bulgarian males, beginning in the mid-1960s. And that "something" was an increase in mortality from heart disease among middle-aged working-class men (Carlson and Tsvetarsky 1992). For women, as seen in table 10.1, life expectancy continued to increase from 1965–67 (72.7 years) to 1989–91 (74.7 years). Therefore, the mortality decline in Bulgaria is chiefly a problem of men.

Besides growing economic and health woes, Bulgarians were fully informed of Gorbachev's reforms through Soviet television and readily available Russian newspapers. Public desires for similar reforms in Bulgaria increased. Zhivkov promised changes but in reality did nothing. A major blunder in attempting to divert public attention from the economic situation in 1989 was Zhivkov's efforts to assimilate Bulgaria's Turkish minority by declaring them "Bulgarian" and canceling their rights as a minority. Some Turks rioted and people were killed by the police in response. Zhivkov recognized his mistake but compounded it by allowing the Turkish population to emigrate, which turned into one of the largest out-migrations of people in modern European history (Glenny 1993). Many of the Turks were skilled industrial workers and farmers and their loss had a serious and immediate impact on the labor force (Holmes 1997). This situation was a major diplomatic embarrassment for the Soviet Union, which was attempting to enhance its own international standing under Gorbachev, and it seriously strained relations with Turkey. A power struggle took place within the Communist Party leadership over whether or not to implement reforms, and Zhivkov was ousted from leadership on 10 November 1989—the same day the Berlin Wall fell. He had ruled for 35 years. As British journalist David Pryce-Jones (1995:297–8) describes the scene:

> On 9 November, in the Politburo, [Petar] Mladenov [the foreign minister] confronted Zhivkov, pressing for his resignation. Evidently, Zhivkov believed that he could prevaricate. Next day at the Central Committee meeting, Prime Minister [Georgi] Atanasov repeated the call to resign and the Central Committee voted to accept it. The scene was filmed, and Zhivkov was shown on the news that day looking shocked to the core at the outcome.

Two months later, with reform communists in power, the Bulgarian Communist Party changed its name to the Bulgarian Socialist Party (BSP). Legislation was passed to end the one-party rule and free multiparty elections were promised for 1990. In March 1990, at roundtable talks with the opposition, an agreement was reached between the socialists and their opponents to appoint multiparty elections for June the same year. The BSP won a majority of seats to the national assembly in the election. However, a videotape of Mladenov saying the army should be called on to send in the tanks after being confronted by an angry, jeering crowd unhappy with his leadership was a bombshell during the elections, forcing his resignation in July (Pryce-Jones 1995). The national assembly elected a member—Zhelyu Zhelev—of the major opposition party, the Union of Democratic Forces (UDF), as president. In 1991 the UDF won a small majority of seats in the national assembly. And in 1992 Zhelev was reelected president by the general population when, for the first time in its history, Bulgaria held direct presidential elections. Reform was moving slowly in Bulgaria, but it was nevertheless underway by 1992 as collective farming was abolished and privatization of housing, shops, and small to medium-sized state businesses was authorized. Disputes continued over the privatization of large state enterprises. Bulgaria had entered a postcommunist phase, even though the ex-communist Bulgarian Socialist Party, which enjoyed strong support in rural areas, remained a powerful political force.

The Postcommunist Period

The dominant initial feature of postcommunism was the continued worsening of the economy. The GDP dropped 12% in 1990 and 23% in 1991, while industrial output fell to 60% of its communist-era value. With the collapse of the Soviet Union, Bulgaria, as noted, lost its major trading partner and has been unable to compensate with significant exports elsewhere. Zhelev, who had been president since 1990, left office in early 1997 as his term ended; he did not stand for re-election. The BSP, which held the majority of seats in the national assembly between 1994 and 1996, received most of the public's blame for the country's economic crisis. The economy had stabilized somewhat in 1995 because of positive results the year before. In 1994 the GDP increased 1%, agreements were reached with creditors on repayment of foreign debts, and unemployment fell to 12.8% from 16.4% in 1993. Inflation, however, increased from 93% to 120%. But the country was unable to capitalize on positive trends because of the slow pace of privatization and the closing of inefficient, money-losing state enterprises. Consequently, in 1996, inflation rose 310% and the value of the Bulgarian currency, the lev, fell from 70 to the dollar to 645. Several banks collapsed and the average wage dropped to $30 dollars a month—the lowest of any country in Europe, including Albania. Many basic goods, like tobacco and fruit, were rationed and the cost of food generally was high. Furthermore, Bulgaria's population was declining as births were failing to keep up with deaths. In 1996, for example, there were 14 deaths per 100,000 persons compared to only 8.7 births.

Thousands of antigovernment demonstrators in Sofia demanded early elections and an end to the worst economic crisis in Eastern Europe since the end of communism. Petar Stoyanov, a member of UDF, was elected president by the people in the fall of 1996 and took office in January 1997. Shortly thereafter, the BSP agreed to hold early parliamentary elections in April; the result was a disaster for the socialists. They won only 57 seats to the 240-seat national assembly, while UDF won a majority of 137 seats and smaller parties acquired the remainder. The new government vowed to ease the economic crisis by providing a swifter transition to a market economy, ending price controls, improving trade, fighting organized crime, privatizing more state-owned enterprises, and creating a currency board required for loans by the International Monetary Fund. A measure requesting membership in NATO was also passed. Time will tell whether these new actions will be successful, but Bulgaria is confronting its problems.

Table 10.2

Mortality Rates for Selected Major Causes of Death for Males and Females, per 100,000 Population, Bulgaria, 1980–1994

Causes of Death	Males			Females		
	1980	1991	1994	1980	1991	1994
All causes	12.1	13.5	15.1	9.8	11.1	11.5
Cancer	1.2	2.1	2.3	1.1	1.4	1.5
Cardiovascular diseases	6.3	7.9	8.8	6.0	7.3	7.7
Stroke	2.7	2.6	—	2.8	2.6	—
Diseases of the respiratory system	1.2	0.8	0.8	0.8	0.5	0.5
Diseases of the digestive system	0.3	0.5	0.6	0.2	0.2	0.2
Accidents and poisoning	0.9	0.9	1.1	0.3	0.3	0.3

SOURCE: Bulgarian National Center of Health Informatics 1995.

One of the most important problems is declining male life expectancy. Referring again to table 10.1, male longevity not only decreased from 68.8 years in 1965–67 to 68 years in 1989–91 but it continued to steadily decline to 67.1 years in 1993–95. Over the last 30 years, Bulgarian male life expectancy has fallen 1.7 years. Female life expectancy, on the other hand, has continued to increase and reached 74.8 years in 1993–95. Table 10.2 shows mortality rates for selected causes of death in Bulgaria for 1980, 1991, and 1994. Deaths from all causes rose for men from 12.1

per 1,000 in 1980 to 15.1 in 1994; deaths for women rose from 9.8 per 1,000 to 11.5 during the same period. The leading cause of death was cardiovascular disease, which increased for men from 6.3 per 1,000 in 1980 to 8.8 in 1994 and from 6 for women in 1980 to 7.7 in 1994. Also shown in table 10.2 are mortality rates for stroke for 1980 and 1991, which were 2.7 and 2.6 per 1,000 respectively for men, and 2.8 and 2.6 for women. These rates are significant because strokes killed a higher percentage of Bulgarians in the 1980s than anywhere else in the world. In 1985, some 58,000 Bulgarians suffered strokes and nearly 24,000 died. Similar but much smaller increases occurred for cancer, respiratory and digestive diseases, and accidents and poisonings. The single most significant killer of Bulgarians is heart disease, which in 1995 caused 63.6% of all deaths. Next, I review the social causes of this situation.

THE SOCIAL DETERMINANTS OF THE DECLINE IN LIFE EXPECTANCY

As in the other former socialist countries, policy, societal stress, and health lifestyles seem to be contributing factors, with health lifestyles the dominant cause of premature male mortality.

Policy

The end of communism brought policy changes to the health care delivery system. One of the first measures in 1990 was to allow patients to choose their own doctors and to authorize doctors to work, with restrictions on the type of care provided, on a fee-for-service basis afterhours. Private practice was authorized as well. By 1995 patients no longer had the option to choose their own individual general practitioner but were required to do so. The primary care doctor, in turn, selected any specialists the patient might need. Choices were limited, however, by having to choose someone from the staff of one's district polyclinic (Popova and Feschieva 1995). Plans were also developed for a compulsory national health insurance system supported by contributions of 6% of wages from employers and 6% from employees. The government-sponsored insurance program was intended to provide a basic level of coverage for everyone, with private insurance available for extra benefits. The unemployed and pensioners were to have coverage paid for by their local government.

However, the national health insurance program has not been implemented, only planned, because of the economic crisis. High unemployment undermined the funding base of employer-employee contributions to the program. In addition, there were major shortages of medical supplies and drugs in the mid-1990s. The amount of the GDP spent on health declined from 5.1% in 1993 to 3.4% in 1997. Moreover, the salaries of state-employed physicians are among the lowest in Eastern Europe, with doctors earning as little as $35 to $100 a month. Bulgaria's health policy has, therefore, not improved the nation's health in any major way in the 1990s. Urban-rural differences in the quality of health care remain, and the system as a whole has not adapted to the rise in chronic illnesses and to changes in society generally (Minev et al. 1990).

However, it is not the health care system that caused the slow decline in male life expectancy. Longevity for females increased in the same health services context in which male life expectancy decreased. Furthermore, there is evidence that Bulgaria has sufficient health care personnel and institutions; there is one doctor per every 335 residents (Popova and Feschieva 1995). Therefore, the ultimate cause of rising male mortality is external to medical practice, even though ineffective treatment contributes to mortality.

Societal Stress

In 1989 the Bulgarian people had great hope for the future. But in 1990 they were facing food shortages and a worsening economy. Many people were fearful about losing their jobs. Some factories closed and unemployment rose. In the mid-1990s economic problems continued, investment declined, and serious inflation persisted. Bulgarians lacked experience in coping with rising unemployment and undoubtedly many people experienced considerable personal stress from their economic situation. However, studies are lacking on the relationship between stress and health during this period. And, although the 1990s have been particularly stressful for Bulgarians, female life expectancy has not declined and the slow downturn in male longevity is the continuation of a gradual, long-term trend over the last 30 years. While stress may be an important causal factor in the lessened male life span, it does not seem to be the primary social determinant.

Health Lifestyles

Evidence supporting a dominant role for health lifestyles in rising male mortality comes from several sources. First, it is very clear that the decline is largely due to increased mortality among middle-aged men from heart disease. For example, between 1980 and 1990, cardiovascular mortality for males increased from 46.4 per 100,000 in the 30–39 age-group to 56.1 per 100,000. In the 40–49 age-group the increase was from 194.5 to 213.6, but the most dramatic upsurge occurred during this period in the 50–59 age-group where the increase was from 486.8 to 742.8. Mortality from cardiovascular diseases declined slightly between 1980 and 1990 for males ages 60 and over (3,809 versus 3,801.4). Mortality increases for women were much more modest. For example, at ages 50 to 59, deaths from cardiovascular diseases increased from 250.4 per 100,000 to 255.9 between 1980 and 1990. So the locus of the downturn in life expectancy is in heart disease among middle-aged males, especially those in their 50s.

In addition, the increased mortality is concentrated among manual workers. In fact, there is a considerable gap between manual and nonmanual workers in mortality. As American demographer Elwood Carlson and his Bulgarian colleague Sergey Tsvetarsky (1992:81) point out, this gap constitutes a dividing line that marks an enduring and important dimension of the social structure and daily life. Carlson and Tsvetarsky (1992:83) conclude that "it is quite close to the truth to say in Bulgaria, virtually all of the increase in working-age male mortality has been concentrated among the manual workers, while nonmanual earners appear to have been largely immune to the worsening mortality trend." Thus, the question that needs to be answered is why has mortality risen so significantly for middle-aged working-class males?

The answer is found in research on health lifestyles. The major work in this area is that of Nevyana Feschieva and her colleagues. In a comparison of health lifestyles in Varna, Bulgaria, and Glasgow and Edinburgh, Scotland, the Bulgarians had significantly worse health lifestyles (Uitenbroek, Kerekovska, and Feschieva 1996). In contrast to the Scots, the Bulgarians smoked significantly more, ate fewer fruits and vegetables, and exercised less. The Scots consumed more alcohol, however. While the results seemed to be related to socioeconomic differences in the development of the three cities—with people in Edinburgh being the healthiest and most affluent, followed by Glasgow, and Varna last—the researchers were not fully satisfied with this explanation. Instead, they suggested it is also necessary to understand the effects of poverty on the individual and the basis upon which individuals make choices. It has, of course, been the central theme of this book that lifestyle choices, even during periods of uncertainty, are mitigated by life chances and tend to fall into routine, predictable, and structured patterns. These patterns are guided by a habitus that channels the health-related behavior down a path that becomes normative for the individual. Consequently, if people drink and smoke too much, eat badly, and do not exercise, these behaviors are norms that have been established through social interaction in relation to the opportunities structured by their society. Bulgarian middle-aged working-class males have suffered a decline in their life span because of their health lifestyle. This is seen in studies showing higher alcohol consumption in this group, as well as a generally low level of participation in other healthy practices concerning diet and smoking (Kerekovska and Feschieva 1995).

As for gender differences, there seems to be little or no leisure-time exercise for either sex; however, men are more likely to exercise than women and consume considerably more alcohol and cigarettes, but women eat more fresh fruits and vegetables (Kerekovska and Feschieva 1995). Alcohol consumption is not as high as in Russia and the style of drinking varies in that most alcohol is consumed at meals. Smoking is perhaps a bigger problem because when socioeconomic status increases, exercise and fruit and vegetable consumption increase as well, but smoking does not decrease. Diet has also been a particular problem for Bulgarians, despite the country's status as a food-producing country, because of high food prices. Between 1991 and 1994 the cost of food rose 239.5%. Milk alone was three times more expensive in the mid-1990s than at the beginning of the decade. Consequently, it is not surprising that the consumption of cereal products, meat, fats, sugar, and milk products decreased between 1989 and 1992 (Sekula, Babinska, and Petrova 1997). Sekula et al. (1997:s64) summarize the current situation in Bulgaria with respect to diet as follows:

> The transition from a centrally planned to a market economy led to many economic problems including the abolition of food subsidies, a decline in agricultural production, a drastic increase in food prices resulting in an increase in the proportion of income spent on food, a significant increase in the rate of unemployment, a decrease in the real incomes of the population, particularly of pensioners, and a decrease of social benefits. These events increased the risk of nutrient deficiencies and unhealthful diets among the Bulgarian population, particularly among high-risk groups.

In sum, Bulgaria has the same overall mortality pattern common to most Eastern Europe on countries in the late twentieth century, originating from the same sources and having the same outcome. Although the decline in male longevity is not as severe as elsewhere, it is a long-term trend that needs to be reversed. But, given Bulgaria's poor economic situation, achieving success in this area is a major challenge.

Chapter 11

East Germany

Of all the former Soviet-bloc countries, only East Germany gave the appearance of avoiding the downturn in male life expectancy. Yet this was not actually the case, as reliable statistics show that the East German state did not entirely escape regional trends, and increases in longevity were significantly slowing over time. Furthermore, the population experienced declining male mortality after the collapse of the communist regime. Had the health and life expectancy of East Germans been better than that of West Germans, the superiority of Soviet-style health care delivery could have been demonstrated. The division of Germany into separate capitalist and socialist states offered the opportunity to evaluate "a natural experiment in history" (Light and Schuller 1986; Volpp 1991). However, by unification, East Germany's health care system was judged a major failure and none of its features were retained (Apelt 1991; Knox 1993; Niehoff, Schneider, and Wetzstein 1992; Volpp 1991). Like Soviet-style health care systems elsewhere in Eastern Europe, the East German approach was becoming increasingly ineffective in coping with heart disease (Knox 1993).

SOCIAL CHANGE

Germany lay in ruins after its defeat in 1945. Neither the victorious Soviet Union nor the Western allies were certain about the future of the country. Stalin expected a communist state to emerge and the Western allies were determined not to allow this to happen in the part of Germany they controlled. By 1946 it was obvious that relations between the Soviets and the West were deteriorating. While the Soviets set about establishing a communist regime in eastern Germany, the Americans and British began rebuilding the West German economy and organizing democratic institutions; in addition, the allies undertook a major currency reform in June 1948 which the Soviets did not accept. The Soviets retaliated by closing off the land access to Berlin, which they occupied jointly with the Americans and the British. And the allies responded by an airlift, which flew supplies into Berlin for 328 days during 1948 and 1949 after which Stalin ended the blockade. Next, the allies promoted the idea of an independent state for their part of Germany and in May 1949 the Federal Republic of Germany was established for western Germany. In response, the German Democratic Republic was founded for the East Germans in the Soviet zone of occupation in October 1949. Cold war competition thus resulted in the establishment of two German states: one in the western alliance and the other in the Soviet bloc, one capitalist and the other Marxist-Leninist. The differences could not be more fundamental. British historian Mary Fulbrook (1993:211–12) provides a concise summary of the relationship between these two countries from 1949 to 1989:

> Although very real, the division of Germany was not conceived as irreversible. The existence of two Germanies only became consolidated in a series of stages: the failure of reunification initiatives in 1952; the incorporation into a range of economic, political, and military alliances in east and west respectively in the course of the 1950s, and the regaining of full sovereignty in 1955; the building of the Berlin Wall in August 1961, when division was literally sealed in concrete, with the closing off of the last means of escape from east to west; the Ostpolitik of the early 1970s, which culminated in mutual recognition in 1972 and entry as full members of the United Nations in 1973; and the development of relations between the two German states in the later 1970s and 1980s, which were distinctively different from relations between any other two separate and sovereign states. The question of German division was then reopened in a startling manner with the East German revolution of autumn 1989 and the opening of the Berlin Wall.

West Germany, aided initially by the Marshall Plan, which provided funds for reconstruction, experienced an "economic miracle" by building one of the strongest and most successful economies in the world. East Germany, for its part, had a Soviet-style economic system imposed on it and rebuilt its industrial base as well. German communists, trained and living in exile in the Soviet Union during the Nazi era, returned with the victorious Soviet army to establish a socialist state which Stalin greeted as a turning point in European history. Stalin, of course, was wrong in this regard as the German Democratic Republic (GDR) collapsed and disappeared from the map of Europe after 40 years of existence. Throughout its existence, East Germany had to fight for survival and lost the struggle in 1989 because so many of its citizens—especially young adults—did not want to live under Communism.

A major confrontation occurred in June 1953 when industrial workers in East Berlin revolted over an increase in work quotas and food prices without a corresponding increase in wages. Strikes involving over 300,000 workers occurred in other major cities in support of the uprising in Berlin. The vast majority of the intelligentsia and other essentially middle-class social strata abstained; the uprising was principally a revolt of industrial workers (Dennis 1985). At least 25 people were killed, over 400 injured, and nearly 1,400 received long-term prison sentences as Soviet troops and tanks were sent into the cities and factories to quell the disorder. The East German government followed with concessions by rescinding the new work quota, increasing minimum wages and pensions, reducing food prices, and increasing the production of consumer goods. The government blamed Western agents for the uprising and the status quo returned to East Germany.

In the meantime, the government had started to collectivize agriculture by moving farmers onto large, state-owned estates. This was a difficult and, for some farmers, an unpopular undertaking. The disruption and confusion induced by this radical change caused agricultural production to fall drastically and several thousand farmers to emigrate to West Germany. Farmers were not the only ones leaving. As border controls tightened, East Germans could easily travel from East Berlin to West Berlin, and from West Berlin they could obtain transportation to West Germany or elsewhere. Between 1949 and 1961, some 4 million East Germans emigrated, of whom 2.7 million passed through West Berlin; by August 1961, when the Berlin Wall sealed the opening, nearly 2,000 East Germans were arriving daily to new lives in the west (Lewis 1987:371). Younger people, skilled workers, and members of the intelligentsia comprised a large majority of the migrants. In order to survive and construct a viable socialist society, the East German government had to stop the hemorrhaging of its population and it chose to do this by imprisoning them behind a wall, adding barbed wire and minefields, and shooting them if necessary for trying to leave. This is a damning indictment of the regime. Erich Honecker, who supervised the construction of the Berlin Wall and the closing of the border with West Germany, became general secretary of the East German Communist Party in 1971. British historian Alexandra Richie (1998:731–2) describes Honecker's background and political outlook as follows:

> The dull, reedy-voiced First Secretary was a true product of the German Communist movement and had dedicated his life to a relentless climb to power. Born in the Saarland in 1912, he had spent his youth in Communist organizations, attending a Youth Cadre school in Moscow in 1930–31 and even spending time in the new industrial city of Magnitogorsk, where he became enamored of Stalinist industrialization of the Soviet Union. In 1935 he was captured by the Nazis and sent to Brandenburg prison, from which he was released in 1945. He always made much of his incarceration, ensuring that his Nazi mug shots appeared in the official version of history; he even released the dissident physicist Robert Havemann from house arrest so that the two could attend the celebration of the thirty-fifth anniversary of liberation from Brandenburg prison together, although the scientist was quietly locked up again after the ceremony. Honecker was genuinely impressed by the Red Army's "liberation" of Germany and the creation of the GDR; he was equally grateful for Brezhnev's backing. His first move was to reaffirm his state's commitment to the Soviets, revising the constitution in 1974 by adding that the GDR would be "forever and irreversibly allied with the Soviet Union."

The early period of communist rule was spent on transforming the society and economy to a socialist model. The property of all former Nazis and war criminals was seized, along with any private estates larger than 100 hectares (247 acres). Agricultural land was reorganized into state farms and peasants sent to work on them. This process was begun in 1952 and virtually completed by 1960. And, except for fruits and vegetables, East Germany was nearly self-sufficient in foodstuffs—although consumer choice and quality was limited (Dennis 1985; Fulbrook 1993). According to Fulbrook (1993:234):

> The contrast between the serried ranks of combine harvesters moving in formation across large collectivised East German fields and the single, often horse-drawn carts visible across the landscape of peasant Poland was highly striking to any visitor in the 1980s. A further quite important source of supply of, for example, eggs, in East Germany came from the small private plots and allotment gardens which were actually encouraged by the state in the 1980s as a supplement to the main collectivized production.

Private ownership in industry was ended fairly quickly and all industrial facilities were confiscated by the central government in the name of the people. An emphasis upon the development of heavy industry followed, with priority given to energy and fuel production, and the manufacture of steel, iron, and chemicals. Consumer goods were not important until the 1970s when highly desired products like television sets and automobiles became more available. The overall economy was centrally planned and coordinated by the East German Politburo. Most of the country's industries were located in the densely populated southern portion of the country around Leipzig, Halle, Karl Marx Stadt (Chemnitz), and Dresden and easily became the most important sector of the economy, accounting for over 45% of the GDP in the 1980s. The main trading partners were the Soviet Union, Eastern Europe, Austria, and West Germany.

According to British historian Mike Dennis (1985), the GDR recognized itself as a "class-like" society; that is, it was not a "class" society because class antagonisms and exploitation had ended but the stage of being a "classless" society had not been fully realized because some class distinctions remained. The largest class in the GDR's classification system was the working class, which comprised 89% of East Germany's 1985 population of 16.6 million people. Both manual and nonmanual workers were included in the working class, with some 62.4% of this stratum considered "core" industrial production workers. Next came the collective farm peasantry (6.8%), followed by various small groups (4.2%), such as self-employed professionals, the intelligentsia, and leading party officials.

Although East Germany achieved considerable economic progress and the highest standard of living in the Soviet bloc, it never came close to overtaking West Germany's quality of life (Dennis 1985; Lewis 1987). As Richie (1998) points out, the East Germans did not measure their success against Albania, but against the images of West Germany that came into their home every night from television. By comparison, the GDR looked rather shabby. And that was the case in reality as large sections of cities like East Berlin, Dresden, and Leipzig were unattractive, run-down, and needed paint and repair. The lack of color midst the grey concrete structures was striking; housing, both old and new, was overcrowded; newer homes and apartments constructed according to socialist styles were unsightly; older homes, some with once attractive exteriors, had shabby and decaying interiors; roads were often in need of repair in towns and cities or unpaved in the countryside; and the highways were the same autobahns constructed by Hitler in the 1930s. People had to wait years for telephones, washing machines, refrigerators, and cars. In 1988 only some 16% of East German households had telephones compared to 93% in West Germany, 66% had washing machines compared to 86%, and 52% had color television sets versus 87% in the western lands (Geisser 1996). Moreover, Richie (1998) explains that the much vaunted East German technology was often based on copies of items manufactured in the West. Many industrial deficiencies were not revealed until the collapse of the regime in 1989 and many of the items manufactured were obsolete by Western standards. Furthermore, Richie (1998:753–4) observes that:

> what economic success the GDR did achieve was purchased at great cost to the environment and to people's health. East German industry was filthy. Chemical and metal processing belched waste into the land, air and water; Bitterfeld, with its large chemical industry, became a byword for pollution, as did Eisleben; its Mansfeld metals complex created enormous slag heaps around the area. Eighty percent of electricity was produced by sulphur-rich brown coal and as power plants had no filters and most homes were heated by coal-burning ovens, tons of sulphur dioxide and dust particles were constantly pumped into the air.

East Germany had some of the worst air pollution in Europe, especially in the so-called "black triangle" coal-mining and industrial areas intersecting with the Polish and Czech borders. Environmental pollution, cheap but not high-quality food, poor living conditions, and intense police-state repression—operating with an army of informers working for the Stasi (East German secret police)—suppressing personal freedom were facts of daily life. It is not surprising that many people wanted change. And that is what happened in 1989 as the widespread discontent in the GDR was transformed into what German sociologist Karl-Dieter Opp (1991; Opp and Gern 1993) called the "spontaneous revolution." He found that three conditions helped bring down the East German government: (1) incentives to protest; (2) positive changes in those incentives; and (3) a high degree of spontaneous cooperation.

The primary incentive for revolt was the deep discontent on the part of the East Germans over their low standard of living and their lack of personal freedom. Other incentives included the growing acceptance of protest as an appropriate norm for behaving toward the government, and the social approval given to protesters by a majority of the population. Thus, there was a high degree of public discontent and readiness to join in protest activities. This readiness was somewhat offset by uncertainty about whether protest could actually bring change and the certainty that the government would fight back. Honecker's government was determined not to adopt the restructuring and openness being tried in the former Soviet Union.

Incentives to protest, however, were energized by the opening of the border between Hungary and Austria in the spring of 1989. East Germans traveling to Hungary could cross to Austria without hindrance and go on to West Germany where they were automatically granted citizenship. Some 30,000 East Germans took this route. In Prague, East Germans climbed over the fence of the West German embassy. Some 12,000 East Germans had gone to Prague and also to Warsaw to escape to the West and were allowed to go by train to West Germany; but they were required to transit through East Germany where Honecker wanted them treated as traitors. En route, however, they were cheered by bystanders, and the train station in Dresden was wrecked from fighting between the police and people trying to get on the trains before they pulled away. The failure of the East German government either to reform or stop the out-migration of so many people increased public willingness to protest.

Thousands of people began to demonstrate, especially in Leipzig and East Berlin. The celebrations for the 40th anniversary of the German Democratic Republic on 7 October 1989 were ruined by counterdemonstrations of masses of people shouting "Freedom!" and "We are the People!" Former soviet premier Mikhail Gorbachev, visiting in East Berlin, personally warned the East German leadership of the consequences facing hard-line regimes that ignored the will of the people. But Honecker rejected Gorbachev's advice. As Richie (1998:823) explains, he was appalled by the changes in Hungary and Poland and by the fact that Gorbachev had allowed it to happen; he was also smug about the fact that East Germany provided a higher standard of living than the Soviet Union; and, finally, he disliked Gorbachev and believed he would soon be removed as the Soviet leader. The dilemma for Honecker was that Gorbachev's reforms were popular among his people and he had always told them to be faithful to Soviet policy. Nevertheless, he ordered live ammunition issued to his security forces and gave them written permission to shoot participants in a large demonstration scheduled for Leipzig on 9 October. This was the "Chinese solution," named after the massacre of demonstrators by the Chinese army in Tiananmen Square in Beijing the previous June.

However, some members of the East German Politburo disagreed over this decision. One of them, Egon Krenz, the chief of security, flew to

Leipzig on 9 October and conferred with local leaders at the home of Kurt Masur, the director of Leipzig's famous symphony orchestra. This group agreed to avoid a potentially explosive situation. That night, when the demonstration was held, the police and security troops withdrew. It became clear to most members of the Politburo that change had to come if the regime was to be saved, and they removed Honecker from power. But removing Honecker was the best the Communist Party could do, and the people were not satisfied (Stokes 1993). Massive demonstrations continued, along with the exodus of up to 200,000 East Germans westward. The new government under Krenz tried to slow the migration by giving East Germans the right to travel abroad for 30 days each after applying at police stations. But this measure was quickly denounced. The demonstrations continued until finally, on 8 November, the Berlin Wall was reopened to allow unrestricted travel to West Berlin. As Angus Roxburgh (1992:158) reported: "On that joyous night, millions of Germans celebrated freedom and the end of the post-war division of Europe." Richie (1998) found the emotional scene at the opening of the Berlin Wall indescribable. People wept, cheered, kissed, hugged, and sprayed each other with champagne and beer. Richie (1998:835) states:

> I remember that night as a kind of dream; the atmosphere was one of giddy excitement and joy but also one of sheer disbelief. After nearly three decades people would be allowed the simple experience of walking from one district to another. The experience was quite banal—one simply walked a few meters past a large, ugly structure and into another district. But it meant so much. Delirious crowds continued to surge across—some in their nightclothes and bedroom slippers; everyone sensed this was a moment that they would savor for the rest of their lives.

Other changes followed rapidly. Public demonstrations made it clear that communism was unacceptable, and the communist leaders supporting Honecker were forced out of office by public pressure. Negotiations between Chancellor Helmut Kohl of West Germany and Gorbachev, in consultation with the United States, France, and Great Britain, removed Soviet objections to the reunification of the two German states (Jarausch 1994). At the end of 1990, the German Democratic Republic was incorporated into the Federal Republic of Germany. The division of the German people was over. But, as Fulbrook (1993:245) observed, the "party was not without its hangover." In the period following reunification, tensions arose between the two groups of Germans. The West Germans had to pay higher taxes to support the development of the new eastern lands, while obsolete industries were closed down and unemployment soared. Furthermore, eastern Germany lost much of its markets in the former Soviet bloc because of economic difficulties among its former trading partners and the requirement to be paid for its goods in (West) German marks. By early 1997, unemployment in eastern Germany reached 21.1% and would have gone higher if the federal government had not paid subsidies for jobs that would not have otherwise existed. The social security of guaranteed jobs and price controls under the communists were gone. East Germans now had to compete in a capitalist economic system. Middle-aged and older persons had no experience with this situation and many people lacked initiative which had been repressed in the former state. To a large extent, East Germany was simply gobbled up by its richer and far more powerful neighbor, and is subject to continuous and radical change as the two areas merge. But eastern Germany is fortunate in having a wealthy sponsor and the prognosis for recovery is excellent; it simply needs time to take effect as the younger generation of East Germans adapts to Western forms of education, politics, and economic activities.

HEALTH AND LIFE EXPECTANCY

The former East German health care delivery system was constructed along Soviet dimensions after 1949, but it was not an exact duplicate of the Semashko model (Knox 1993; Marrée and Groenewegen 1997). Health care was not exclusively financed directly out of the budget of the central government; rather, all East Germans were covered by social insurance. About 85% of the population was covered by the Sozialversicherung (SV) fund and the other 15% (civil servants, the self-employed, farmers in cooperatives, and their dependents) by the Deutsche Versicherungsanstalt (DVA). This system was supported by the contributions of employers and employees, with employees paying 10% of their wages up to a maximum of 60 East German marks a month. This contribution covered not only health care, but pension and sick leave payments. The state supplemented the social insurance funds because employer-employee contributions were not sufficient to cover all expenses, but the bulk of health care was financed through insurance. Health care was free to patients. Furthermore, East Germans had free choice of physicians, which was not usually the case in other former socialist countries. And about 13% of all hospitals, typically the better equipped and maintained, were owned by churches. Thus, the GDR's health system retained many aspects of its precommunist period which dated from Bismarck's reforms in Imperial Germany in 1889.

At that time, Bismarck established a program of social insurance based on three principal components: (1) compulsory health insurance, (2) free health services, and (3) sick leave benefits. Bismarck's welfare measures rank among his greatest political accomplishments. They were also an attempt to defuse the demands of the working class for political and social rights by providing them with health care linking them to the state rather than to labor unions or socialist political parties. Bismarck was forced to make some concessions by allowing intermediate institutions between the government and the people to assume fiscal responsibility for the delivery of services. Under this model, the government does not play a major role in the financing of health services; rather, its primary role is one of administration, regulation, and supervision. According to American medical sociologist Donald Light (1986; Light and Schuller 1986), this form of health service organization is one of corporatism and represents a unique contribution by Germany to the provision of health care. Corporatism, in the German context, consists of: (1) compulsory membership on the part of the population in a national health plan; and (2) a set of institutions situated between the government and its citizens with the authority to manage health care delivery and acquire, negotiate, and pay for health services under government auspices. This is the system used in the former West Germany and the unified German state today. However, the East German government took direct control over its system by establishing a hierarchy of hospitals and polyclinics reporting to the Ministry of Health, taking over ownership of most health care facilities, making physicians and health care workers employees of the state, and setting goals and priorities. The social insurance funds were strictly limited to the financing of services and had no managing or negotiating role.

In 1987–88, the GDR spent 5.2% of its GDP on health, which was relatively high among the former socialist countries but insufficient to meet the needs of the population. Doctors and nurses were not especially well paid, though they were paid higher than elsewhere in the Soviet bloc and could work privately after their usual working hours for the state had ended. The physical condition of numerous hospitals and polyclinics was poor and both modern equipment and medical supplies were in short supply, especially toward the end of the regime. The average age of an East German hospital in 1988 was more than 60 years. Many had severe structural problems like leaking roofs, outmoded electrical systems, dysfunctional heating systems, and inadequate sewage and sanitation facilities (Knox 1993:259). Furthermore, East Germany had a highly stratified system of health care delivery which divided resources unevenly (Apelt 1991). There were 14 separate health systems, organized to provide services to top party officials and diplomats, the police, the army, the secret police, construction workers, uranium miners, transportation workers, various other industrial workers, members of scientific academies, university staffs, victims of fascism, elite athletes, church-run systems, and the public health system (Volpp 1991). At the top end of the health care system were clinics for the political elite equipped with the latest and best technology and few patients per physician; at the bottom end was the public health system, which was the least supported, was overcrowded with patients, and featured long waits for specialized services.

> The under-provision of patients in the public system could not be compensated by over-provision in elite systems because of the impermeability of the systems. Each was based in a different ministry, and the very existence of the other health care systems was a secret to many. These were closed systems for political, not medical reasons. . . . The differences are, however, readily visible and are confirmed by people at every level of the system, leaving little doubt that class medicine was, in fact, the reality in the GDR. (Volpp 1991:6)

It is ironic that a social system designed to promote political, economic, and social equality would be so unequal in the provision of such a basic human need as health care, but that was indeed the case. With the collapse of the GDR and its reunification with West Germany, the East German system was abandoned. West Germany's social insurance funds, some 1,317 in number and mostly organized along occupational lines, were authorized to provide coverage in the new lands (*neue Länder*) and East German physicians literally rushed to set up private practices since state paychecks suddenly stopped. West German physician groups set up workshops throughout the east to show local doctors how to make the transition to an office-based private practice. "East German medicine," states American journalist Richard Knox (1993:270), "was transformed in the space of two years from an almost entirely salaried, state-run enterprise to an entirely private and overwhelmingly free-for-service model."

In the new Western system, social insurance plans issue certificates to members and their dependents which are presented to physicians when services are rendered. The physician then submits the certificate to his or her association of registered doctors which all physicians are required to join. Payment is made to the physician through the association according to a fee schedule agreed upon by the association and the health insurance plan. Hospital fees and payments are handled in the same manner (Lassey, Lassey, and Jinks 1997). Health care is free to the patient and is financed by contributions to the social insurance funds of approximately 12.9% of an employee's wages, with half paid by the employee and half by the employer. Pensioners, the disabled, and the unemployed are supported by the government. Approximately 90% of all Germans participate in the nation's health insurance program. The remainder consists generally of civil servants, the self-employed, and white-collar workers with yearly incomes above the government ceiling (about $45,600 in the west and $35,400 in the east) who voluntarily join the state plan or take out private health insurance. Hospitals operate on budgets negotiated between their associations and the social insurance funds.

Table 11.1

Life Expectancy in East and West Germany, 1950–1995

East			West		
Year	Male	Female	Year	Male	Female
1950	65.1	69.1	1950	64.6	68.5
1960	67.3	72.2	1960	66.7	71.9
1970	68.1	73.3	1969–71	67.3	73.6
1976	68.8	74.4	1975–77	68.6	75.2
1981	69.0	74.8	1980–82	70.2	76.9
1986–87	69.8	75.8	1985–87	71.8	78.4
1988–89	70.0	76.2	1988–90	72.6	79.0
1991–93	69.9	77.2	1991–93	73.1	79.5
1992–94	70.3	77.7	1992–94	73.4	80.0
1993–95	70.7	78.2	1993–95	73.5	79.8

SOURCE: Statisches Bundesamt 1995.

Despite the general quality of health services and more severe environmental pollution in the GDR, East German life expectancy was longer than that of West Germans in the early 1970s. As shown in table 11.1, in 1970 East German males lived 68.1 years on average compared to 67.3 years for West German males in 1969–71. But the advantage was both slight (0.8 years) and temporary. During the nearly 20 years between 1970 and 1988–89, East German male longevity increased only 1.9 years compared to 5.3 years for West German males. Table 11.1 shows that life expectancy for East German males then declined, in the aftermath of communism's fall, from 70 years in 1988–89 to 69.9 years in 1991–93. Following this slight dip, male life expectancy in East Germany recovered to a high of 70.7 years in 1993–95, in comparison to 73.5 years in West Germany. For West German females life expectancy increased from 73.6 years in 1969–71 to 79.8 years (allowing for a small decrease of 0.2 years in 1992–94) in 1993–95; the life span of East German females increased from 73.3 years to 78.2 during this same period.

Figure 11.1

Life Expectancy, Eastern and Western Germany by Sex, 1932–1995

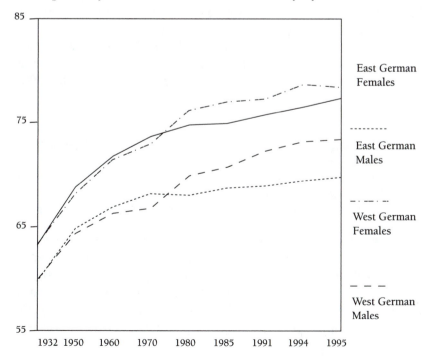

The life expectancy patterns for men and women in both sections of Germany between 1932 and 1995 are depicted in figure 11.1. As shown, both East German men and women outlived their Western counterparts until the 1970s when the West Germans moved ahead to stay. The upward movement of West German females is particularly striking. Also of interest in figure 11.1 is the generally flat profile shown for East German men beginning in 1970. Although these men did not suffer the massive declines in life expectancy seen in other former socialist countries, their longevity was only somewhat better than stagnant. So, the question again is, why have males in a socialist country fared relatively poorly in comparison to females in the same country and to both sexes in a Western country? Once again I turn to a discussion of policy, societal stress, and health lifestyles.

Policy

In many respects, as Jörgen Marrée and Peter Groenewegen (1997:35) point out, the former East German health care system was the most "Western" of the former Soviet-bloc countries. In a comparison of the health situation in East and West Germany two years after the opening of the Berlin Wall, German sociologists Günther Lüschen and Peter Apelt found that East Germany was rapidly adopting the West German health care system, although certain conditions and the general state of health were still linked to the time when the two systems were separate. Lüschen and Apelt (1992:14) found more similarities than differences and commented that:

> a strong impression prevails that the two systems because of their joint history, strong mutual identification, social as well as family exchanges have a strong cultural identity; and this may indicate that the two systems in terms of their health culture were not so far apart after all. It should also be mentioned that the communist regime left much of the health care system untouched and provided physicians with considerable privileges.

In a subsequent study, Lüschen and his colleagues (Lüschen, Niemann, and Apelt 1997) found that, in terms of organization, the most distinct feature of East German health care was the introduction of central state control into the system. Thus, collective forms of care under a centralized state-run system were favored in the GDR over private practice. It did enjoy some success with respect to the lowering of infant mortality which fell from 17 deaths per 1,000 infants in 1960 to 11.1 in 1990, along with the eradication of communicable diseases. But the system was not considered innovative by its clients and it developed a reputation for substandard technology and drugs. Moreover, measures to cope with heart disease were ineffective as the life spans of middle-aged men in particular were shortened (Eberstadt 1994). On balance, it is clear that the system of socialist care in East Germany was in many respects less effective than that of West Germany (Lüschen et al. 1997). East German health policy was intended to provide for the needs of the population and demonstrate socialist superiority over the West. It failed in this regard, but there is no evidence showing policy to be the most important cause of the relatively stagnant life expectancy of East Germany's male population.

Societal Stress

The role of stress in retarding life expectancy in East Germany is not fully known because of a lack of data. One exception is a study by German researchers B. Häussler, Elke Hempel, and P. Reschke (1995), who investigated the decline in East German male longevity after the fall of the Berlin Wall in 1989. A variety of data were used to calculate standardized mortality ratios and differences between East and West were broken down by age-groups. The principal finding was that the life expectancy of East German men declined in 1990 by 0.9 years and did not recover to the 1989 level until 1992. In their calculation, male life expectancy was 70.1 years in 1989, which fell to 69.2 in 1990 and then rose to 69.4 and 70 in 1991 and 1992 respectively. This result was due entirely to an increase in mortality for men under age 65; heart disease and cirrhosis of the liver were the leading causes of death for men between the ages of 45 and 65. Häussler et al. suggest that their findings can be interpreted as showing that the political and social upheaval surrounding the fall of the Berlin Wall produced considerable stress for the men, but not for the women, who were apparently able to better adjust to the situation.

This is an interesting finding because even though East German male longevity was not moving upward very rapidly, the only period in which it actually declined (although it was a relatively small decrease) was after the collapse of communism. However, why would East German women, who were represented in large numbers in the workforce and suffered many of the same strains concerning their job situation when communism ended, not be affected as much as men? This question remains unanswered. German public health researchers and demographers L. Heinemann, R. Dinkel, and E. Görtler (1996), who focused not on the 1989–92 period but on long-term life expectancy trends from 1950 until the early 1990s, concluded that the growing gap between East and West Germany that emerged in the 1970s was largely due to social factors, namely health lifestyles. Heinemann et al. found, for instance, that during the 1960s and 1970s blood pressure and cholesterol levels were significantly increasing in East Germany in comparison to West Germany. West Germany also had more favorable social trends in the form of higher levels of education and a lower proportion of people in the working class, who show themselves to be particularly susceptible to heart disease.

If poor health lifestyles were slowing increases in East German male life expectancy for over 20 years, the societal stress associated with the extreme change in their society may have triggered early deaths among men who were already unhealthy and vulnerable to stress due to their lifestyle practices. Societal stress may, therefore, have played an important role in rising male mortality at a time of significant social upheaval, but stress may not have been the ultimate cause of the vulnerability to its effects. Health lifestyles, not stress, may have been the most significant and underlying determinant of the premature male deaths. This circumstance would help explain the gender difference in mortality.

Health Lifestyles

While there is not an abundance of research on health lifestyles in East Germany, the previously discussed Heinemann et al. (1996) study provided strong evidence of the adverse effects of long-term health lifestyle practices in promoting greater cardiovascular mortality in East Germany as opposed to West Germany. "Whereas," concluded Heinemann et al. (1996:15), "migration, environmental pollution, and health-care differences accounted for only a small part of the gap [between East and West Germany], evidence emerged that lifestyle and social patterns may have caused the less favourable trend in cardiovascular disease." Other comparative data show that the prevalence of heart disease is indeed greater in East Germany than West Germany, with East German males showing higher levels of cigarette smoking, hypertension, cholesterol, and obesity (Häussler et al. 1995; Heinemann, Barth, and Hoffmeister 1995;

Helmert, Mielck, and Classen 1992; Knox 1993; Lüschen et al. 1997). East German females showed a similar pattern except for less smoking. One result is an age-adjusted mortality rate from heart disease in 1988 that was 40% higher for males and 60% higher for females in East Germany as compared to West Germany (Knox 1993).

Other research suggests that East Germans were less likely to exercise and more likely to consume hard liquor than West Germans (Lüschen, Apelt, and Kunz 1993). The East Germans also had a less healthy diet than the West Germans. In East Germany the consumption of milk, vegetable oil, fresh vegetables, and fruit was much lower than in West German, and the intake of sausages and butter was much higher (Thiel and Heinemann 1996). Consequently, the caloric intake in East Germany was higher in fat and lower in carbohydrates. A key difference in the healthier lifestyles found in West Germany may be education, in that the West Germans had a higher overall level of education, and people who are well educated are generally the best informed about the merits of a healthy lifestyle (Heinemann et al. 1996; Lüschen and Apelt 1992). Manual workers and those persons at the bottom of the social scale had the least healthy lifestyles in East Germany (Heinemann et al. 1996).

In sum, it appears that policy and stress are important factors in determining the life expectancy pattern of East German males, but these factors affected all men and women alike. Yet it was the middle-aged working-class male who was affected much more than anyone else, and the reasons for this situation originate in the health lifestyle of this group. This seems to be especially demonstrated in the fact that West German and American men generally showed similar and relatively positive health lifestyle trends involving exercise, diet, smoking, and alcohol use in the mid-1980s (Cockerham, Kunz, and Lueschen 1988). During the same time, longevity was increasing much faster for West German and American males than it was for East German males. Like their socialist colleagues elsewhere in the Soviet bloc, middle-aged working-class East German males ate fatty diets, drank and smoked too much, and did not exercise; as a consequence, they developed cardiovascular problems at earlier ages and died much sooner. Enough of this pattern of behavior existed to significantly slow increases in their life expectancy.

Chapter 12

Conclusion

Health care is a commodity in the modern world; that is, it is something to be purchased despite its status as a basic social right in European societies. The capitalist approach was to establish a fee-for-service system. National health insurance programs, based largely on employee-employer contributions and reinforced by tax revenues, paid the costs. The care itself was generally free for patients. The socialist approach, conversely, was to co-opt health care as a state commodity, paid for out of the central government's budget and provided as a free social benefit to the people. Neither system has worked perfectly, but it is clear from the discussion in this book that the socialist system did not deliver on its promise and the capitalist system, despite its many inequities, did. Western European populations rank among the very healthiest in the world; the former socialist countries generally rank toward the bottom of industrialized nations in health.

The evolution of this situation is rooted in the European concept of the welfare state. During the early twentieth century, when European society was still grounded in imperialism and competition for political, economic, and military domination, many governments and industrialists desired healthy populations whose productivity could be translated into economic power. Greater economic power, in turn, meant greater political and military power, as well as securing a higher standard of living for the nation and increased profits from trade and manufacturing. In some capitalist countries, providing state-sponsored welfare was also a means to reduce discontent and the threat of revolution from the working class. Social insurance programs were essentially designed to protect the income of workers when sick, disabled, unemployed, or old. The existing private health insurance and pension plans were often unable to adequately meet the needs of the entire population, especially of those individuals who were unable to afford coverage. It therefore fell to national governments to take greater responsibility for the welfare of the governed.

Initially, social insurance was provided by many of the European governments only to wage earners below a certain income level, but gradually benefits were extended to all or most of the population in capitalist countries. According to British sociologist T. H. Marshall (1964), the advent of the welfare state in the West was a culmination of processes that began in the eighteenth century. Marshall points out that the establishment of the welfare state is a late phase in an evolution of citizens' rights in Western society. To *civil* rights (gained in the eighteenth century), like freedom of speech and equality before the law, and *political* rights (acquired in the late eighteenth and the nineteenth centuries), such as the right to vote and participate in the exercise of government, were added the *social* rights (achieved in the late nineteenth and twentieth centuries) of protection from economic insecurity and provision of at least a marginal level of subsistence. The latter includes health care. The emergence of these various rights of citizenship, all promoting equality, states Marshall, is a paradox, because they came during the same historical period as the rise of capitalism, which is a system of inequality. Inequality in the capitalist system stems from the fact that it is based on private ownership of property and the gearing of economic activity to profit in the marketplace. Individuals are not equal in the amount of property they own or acquire, in their position in relation to the production of goods and services, and in the amount of profits (or losses) they derive from their work. As American sociologist John Myles (1984:30) comments, "This marriage between a protective state and a capitalist economy was a union of opposites, for it required an accommodation between two opposing logics of distribution—one that attached rights to the possession of *property* and another that attached rights to *persons* in their capacity as citizens."

Essentially, what had happened, in Marshall's (1964) view, was a "war" between the rights of citizenship, considered inherent in a democratic society by the general populace, and the capitalist class system. In the modern welfare state individual rights of citizenship, not ownership of property, emerged as the basis for political representation and entitlement to social programs like national health insurance. As the system evolved in Western Europe, health care benefits were not based on the incomes of individuals but on their status as citizens (or qualified residents), which meant that *everyone* was entitled to a basic level of health care. If there was some discrimination in the system, then typically the affluent, as in the case of Germany and elsewhere, were more on their own in obtaining health coverage; the poor, disabled, and unemployed were guaranteed care. And, in a national health insurance system in Western Europe, socially and economically disadvantaged persons participated in the mainstream health care delivery system—not in some inferior and poorly funded program that marked their social status as less than that of others.

Consequently, patterns of social stratification in relation to health services utilization in Western Europe usually do not differ significantly, except that the lower social strata tend to have the worst health and seek care from physicians the most (Lüschen et al. 1995). Although there are class differences in mortality, the social welfare provisions reflected in health benefits are based on considerations of equity, and social inequality is not an inherent part of the pattern of health care. But health care is still a commodity and in the Western European case national health insurance programs backed by the state guarantee its availability to the individual. Patients have choices of physicians and hospitals and payments for their services are made by third parties—usually health insurance funds supplemented by the state.

This situation strongly contrasts with the approach used in the former socialist countries. Under socialism, the state owned the health care system and providers were government employees. Health care itself was a state commodity provided for free to citizens as a product of socialism. In return, citizens were to be suitably grateful and loyal to the state for keeping them healthy. Officially, there were no insurance payments, deductions from wages, or out-of-pocket costs. Unofficially, there were under-the-table payments to providers by individuals seeking some consideration beyond that typically extended in a collective system.

There were several problems with this arrangement. First, the socialist states did not adequately finance the provision of health care. As discussed earlier in this book, the health sector was regarded as "nonproductive" in that it did not contribute to the state's coffers; it took money rather than produced money. Furthermore, it was not as important in projecting state power as heavy industry, collectivized agriculture, and the military were. When budgets were tight and money in short supply, health care received what was left (the so-called "residue" principle). Therefore, health services in the former Soviet bloc were never a priority, nor ever funded sufficiently by the state. Poor-quality service signified poor-quality care for the bulk of the population. Whereas this policy did not cause the massive increase in male heart disease, it undoubtedly produced deaths that could have been avoided if better medical resources had been provided.

Second, despite its failure to provide quality health care to the population, the socialist state assumed responsibility for everyone's health. This had an extremely negative effect on individuals who placed responsibility for their health in the hands of a state system that could not be adequately responsible because of a lack of resources and initiative. Moreover, this induced a social-psychological dependence on the state which promoted a lack of personal responsibility on the part of the individual. Consequently, certain people, especially middle-aged working-class males, felt free to engage in unhealthy lifestyle practices because they assumed the state would take care of them. The behaviors that supported these practices were grounded in group norms for social interaction. Thus, bad health lifestyle practices became normative for these men and in time constituted what Pierre Bourdieu (1984) calls a habitus—a structured structure operating as a structuring structure that predisposes the person to follow a particular line of behavior as opposed to others that might be chosen. As a set of predispositions to act in a certain way, the habitus is a mental scheme or organized framework of perceptions that guides and evaluates choices. These perceptions are developed, shaped, and maintained in memory and habits through socialization, experience, and the reality of class circumstances. The habitus "only exists inasmuch as it is 'inside the heads' of actors" (Jenkins 1992:75) and is a mental process that mediates between the interests of individuals and groups on one side and the structural context of social practices on the other. While the behavior selected may be contrary to normative expectations, behavioral choices are typically compatible with the norms of a particular group, class, or larger society; therefore, people usually act in predictable and habitual ways.

The habitus of individuals emerges from their conditions of living and their relative position within the social structure of those conditions. People who share the same living conditions and relative social positions tend to develop the same habitus and social practices. "These practices," claims Bourdieu (1977:78), "can be accounted for only by relating the objective *structure* defining the social conditions of the production of the habitus which engendered them to the conditions in which this habitus is operating, that is, to the *conjuncture* which, short of a radical transformation, represents a particular state of this structure." Therefore, members of a particular social class share a similar class habitus and out-look. Bourdieu explains that while it is impossible that all members of a particular social class will have had the same exact experiences, it is cer-tain that people in the same class are more likely than people in another class to have experienced situations most frequent for members of that class. This circumstance creates the basis for a class-oriented habitus. Even though people may bring their own "personal style" to their habi-tus and practices, differences in each individual's system of dispositions may be seen as variant of a particular class habitus that is commonly shared. Consequently, Bourdieu (1977:95) finds that "because the habi-tus is an endless capacity to engender products—thoughts, perceptions, expressions, actions—whose limits are set by the historically and social-ly situated conditions of its production, the conditioned and conditional freedom it secures is as remote from a creation of unpredictable novelty as it is from a simple reproduction of the initial conditionings." The result is that people tend to follow behavioral pathways that are consistent with their class-based habitus, even though some personal nuances may occur.

Bourdieu (1984:171) also observes that the social practices produced by a class habitus constitute a lifestyle that is operationalized in the fol-lowing manner: (1) objective living conditions combine with relative posi-tions in the social structure to produce (2) a habitus that (3) consists of a system of schemes with the capacity to generate classifiable practices and works, and (4) a system of schemes of perception and appreciation ("taste"), which between them (5) produce classifiable practices and works, resulting in (6) a particular lifestyle. Bourdieu's theoretical per-spective is relevant for the health outcomes of middle-aged working-class men in the former socialist countries because it explains the process by which the habitus of this group evolved into a highly negative health lifestyle. The (1) poor living conditions of Soviet-bloc manual workers and their relatively low (despite their exalted place in socialist ideology) and powerless position in the social structure produced (2) a habitus with (3) a system of schemes having the tendency to produce unhealthy prac-tices and (4) a system of schemes of perception and appreciation of those practices (such as heavy drinking and smoking, disregard for diet, and rejection of exercise) which (5) produced these practices and resulted in (6) a lifestyle that promoted heart disease, accidents, and other health problems leading to a shortened life. Dependence and trust in a faltering state health care delivery system corrupted by the payment of gratuities and a hierarchical system of health facilities favoring the elite, unfortu-nately added another structural dimension to the habitus—a false sense of security. Medical treatment and health policies in the respective countries could not compensate for an unhealthy lifestyle and stress was a likely contributing factor to this negative way of living. Ultimately, the cause of the downturn in life expectancy can be traced to lifestyle.

German sociological theorist Richard Münch (1993) joins others (Alexander 1995) in criticizing Bourdieu's analysis as overdeterministic. In their view, Bourdieu's work overemphasizes the power of structure and seems—despite Bourdieu's objections—to relegate the individual to a relatively passive role in both the selection of behavior and the capacity to induce social change. Agency is not missing, just marginalized. Consequently, praxis seems dominated by structure. According to Münch (1993:153–4), "Bourdieu has a structural bias and therefore sees the relationship too one-sidedly, from structure to habitus to praxis to life-styles, and not in the converse direction, from life-styles to praxis to habitus and to structure." This is an important observation because it raises the question: How does structural change occur? The origin of structural change could reside in lifestyles but this potential is not specified in Bourdieu's work. However, Bourdieu's theory fits the experience of the former socialist societies because their structures *were* overly deterministic and there was little possibility for social change until the end of socialism. The potential for the emergence of a lifestyle constructed by agency and having the capacity to alter structure through a reverse feedback process in such a society was nil. The communist system of centralized control was too rigid and inflexible to permit change from below. Change could only come from the top, which was impossible until Gorbachev and his effort to induce change shattered the brittle structure supporting the Soviet state. So, whereas Bourdieu's work may not be fully applicable to all social scenarios, his strong emphasis on structure captures the lack of freedom and the limited range of individual lifestyle choices under socialism.

As noted briefly in the chapter on Bulgaria, the central theme of this book is that lifestyle choices, even during periods of postmodern change and uncertainty, are mitigated by life chances and tend to fall into particular patterns. Therefore, if middle-aged working-class men in the former socialist countries ate fatty foods, drank and smoked too much, and did not exercise, these behaviors were norms established through group interaction, *structured* by the opportunities provided by society, and internalized by these men's habitus. In the former Soviet-bloc societies there was not much opportunity to make choices promoting a healthy lifestyle. Alcohol was usually cheap and cigarettes were readily available. Food choices were severely limited in quality and availability, and group norms promoting leisure-time exercise were absent. In this type of situation, structure (chance), not agency (choice), becomes the dominant factor when a habitus structured to operate in these conditions is added. While one might argue there is always a choice, there are times when opportunities and choices are so severely limited that group norms can become punishing, as seen in the outcome of greater heart disease and other mortality-producing illnesses from poor lifestyle practices.

The objective of this book is to uncover the primary social determinants of the downturn in life expectancy in Russia and Eastern Europe. The principal victims, as noted, of this public health disaster are working-class males, primarily manual workers, who succumb largely to heart disease in middle age. Policy, societal stress, and health lifestyles appear to be the major potential sources of adverse male health in the region and each is found to make an important contribution to rising male mortality. But, ultimately, the thesis of this book is that negative health lifestyles are the primary social determinant of the decline in life expectancy. The structure surrounding the daily life of middle-aged working-class males both limited and shaped choices to the extent that their lifestyle led to early deaths. This development was bound up in the larger structure of socialist societies, with their centralized planning and control systems that determined the opportunities and quality of life for their citizens. The needs of the state came first and the state never reached a position of improving the life of the individual; rather, the party elite was able to corrupt the system for their own ends, while the average person in a European socialist country fared poorly, not only in material goods and health, but in personal freedom and initiative.

A major undertaking today in the region should be the implementation of extensive public education programs to help people realize the necessity of living healthier lifestyles. There are many other needs as well: *well-trained* health care providers, improved and updated facilities and technology, national health insurance coverage for the entire population, a greater annual share of the GDP devoted to health, the provision on a large scale of healthy foods, opportunities for leisure-time exercise, and the public negation of the unhealthy effects of alcohol consumption and smoking. The introduction of all these measures, along with the development of individual responsibility for health on a massive scale, are needed to correct unhealthy lifestyle practices and reverse the downward trend in life expectancy in the former socialist countries.

Appendix

Correlation Coefficient, Means, and Standardized Deviations (N = 8,402)

	1	2	3	4	5	6	7	8	9	10	11	12	13
1. Alcohol	1.00												
2. Smoking	.20												
3. Exercise	.06	.01											
4. Fat intake	.08	.04	.06										
5. Health status	.13	.13	.16	.17									
6. Life satisfaction	.06	.00	.13	.11	.19								
7. Male	.15	.55	.11	.07	.20	.06							
8. Age	-.16	-.19	-.23	-.12	-.52	-.14	-.12						
9. Education	.19	-.01	.05	.15	.14	.07	-.01	-.14					
10. Income	.07	.02	.06	.07	.03	.11	.00	-.01	.09				
11. Urban	.07	.02	.10	.06	.05	.08	-.00	-.05	.21	.04			
12. Married	.15	.09	-.12	.07	.03	.00	.15	.04	.25	.01	-.01		
13. Employed	.25	.18	.00	.12	.23	.04	.17	-.24	.34	.07	.09	.25	
Mean	2.50	.31	.44	32.41	3.11	2.24	.44	44.71	2.18	372751	.74	.63	.51
SD	2.47	.46	1.03	10.09	.78	1.09	.50	18.24	1.86	657596	.44	.48	.50

References

Abel, Thomas. 1991. Measuring Health Lifestyles in a Comparative Analysis: Theoretical Issues and Empirical Findings. *Social Science and Medicine* 32:899–908.

Abel, Thomas, and William C. Cockerham. 1993. Lifestyle or Lebensführung? Critical Remarks on the Mistranslation of Weber's "Class, Status, Party." *Sociological Quarterly* 34:551–6.

Adevi, O., G. Chellaraj, E. Goldstein, A. Preker, and D. Ringold. 1997. Health Status During the Transition in Central and Eastern Europe: Development in Reverse? *Health Policy and Planning* 12:132–45.

Adler, Nancy E., Thomas Boyce, Margaret A. Chesney, Sheldon Cohen, Susan Folkman, Robert L. Kahn, and S. Leonard Syme. 1994. Socioeconomic Status and Health: The Challenge of the Gradient. *American Psychologist* 49:15–24.

Alexander, Jeffrey C. 1987. The Dialetic of Individuation and Domination: Weber's Rationalization Theory and Beyond. Pp. 185–206 in Max Weber, *Rationality and Modernism*, edited by S. Whimster and S. Lash. London: Allen and Unwin.

———. 1995. *Fin de siècle Social Theory*. London: Verso.

Anderson, Barbara A., and Brian D. Silver. 1990. Trends in Mortality of the Soviet Population. *Soviet Economy* 3:191–251.

Andreev, Y. M. 1990. Prodolzhiitelnost zhizni i prichini smerti v SSSR [Life expectancy and causes of death in the U.S.S.R.]. Pp. 90–116 in *Demograficheskiye Processi v SSSR*. Moscow: Nauka.

Antal, László Z. 1994. *Causes of High Mortality Rate in the Former Socialist Countries*. Budapest: Hungarian Academy of Sciences.

Apelt, Peter. 1991. Gleichheit und Ungleichheit im Gesundheitswesen der DDR [Equality and inequality in health systems in the German Democratic Republic]. *Mensch Medizin Gesellschaft* 16:27–33.

Åslund, Anders. 1995. *How Russia Became a Market Economy*. Washington, D.C.: Brookings Institute.

Báska, T., and S. Straka. 1995. Je sucasny trend umrtnosti na kardiovaskularne ochorenia v Slovenskej republike dovodom k optimizu? [Is the present trend in cardiovascular disease mortality in the Slovak Republic a reason for optimism?]. *Epidemiologie, Mikrobiologie, Immunologie* 44:177–9.

Barr, Donald A., and Mark G. Field. 1996. The Current State of Health Care in the Former Soviet Union: Implications for Health Care Policy and Reform. *American Journal of Public Health* 86:307–12.

Baudrillard, Jean. 1988. *Selected Writings*. Edited by M. Poster. Stanford, Calif.: Stanford University Press.

Bauman, Zygmunt. 1992. *Intimations of Postmodernity*. London: Routledge.

Beck, Ulrich. 1992. *Risk Society*. Translated by M. Ritter. London: Sage.

———. 1994. The Reinvention of Politics: Towards a Theory of Reflexive Modernization. Pp. 1–55 in *Reflexive Modernization*, by Ulrich Beck, Anthony Giddens, and Scott Lash. Stanford, Calif: Stanford University Press.

Beck, Ulrich, Anthony Giddens, and Scott Lash. 1994. *Reflexive Modernization*. Stanford, Calif.: Stanford University Press.

Bejnarowicz, Janusz. 1994. Changes in Poles' Health Status and in its Determinants (in Polish). *Health Promotion, Social Sciences and Medicine* 1(2): 9–36.

Beliaev, E. N. 1996. Monitoring pitaniia i kachestva pishchevykh produktov v sisteme sotsial'no-gigienicheskogo monitoringa v Rossiiskoi Federatsii [Monitoring nutrition and the quality of the food products in the social-hygiene monitoring system in the Russian Federation]. *Voprosy Pitaniia* 3:3–8.

Bell, Daniel. 1991. Values and the Future in Marx and Marxism. *Futures* (March):146-62.

Bendix, Reinhard. 1960. *Max Weber: An Intellectual Portrait*. New York: Doubleday.

Bertens, Hans. 1995. *The Idea of the Postmodern: A History*. London: Routledge.

Best, Steven, and Douglas Kellner. 1991. *Postmodern Theory: Critical Interrogations*. New York: Guilford Press.

Biro, G. 1996. Cardiovascular Risk Factors Distribution in Hungarian Adults. *Acta Cardiologica* 51:113–28.

Biro, G., M. Antal, and G. Zajkas. 1996. Nutrition Survey of the Hungarian Population in a Randomized Trial Between 1992–1994. *European Journal of Clinical Nutrition* 50:201–8.

Blaxter, Mildred. 1990. *Health and Lifestyles*. London: Routledge.

Bobák, Martin, Zdenka Škodová, Zbynek Píša, Rudolf Poledne, and Michael Marmot. 1997. Political Changes and Trends in Cardiovascular Risk Factors in the Czech Republic, 1985–92. *Journal of Epidemiology and Community Health* 51:272-7.

Bocock, Robert. 1993. *Consumption*. London: Routledge.

Bojan, Ferenc, Piroska Hajdu, and Eva Belicza. 1991. Avoidable Mortality. Is It an Indicator of Quality of Medical Care in Eastern European Countries? *Quality Assurance in Health Care* 3:191–203.

———. 1993. Regional Differences in Avoidable Mortality in Europe. Pp. 125–39 in *Europe Without Frontiers The Implications for Health*, edited by C. Normand and P. Vaughan. Chichester, U.K.: Wiley.

Borissov, Vesselin, and Tom Rathwell. 1996. Health Care Reforms in Bulgaria: An Initial Appraisal. *Social Science and Medicine* 42:1501–10.

Bottomore, Tom. 1984. *Sociology and Socialism*. Brighton, U.K.: Wheatsheaf.

Bourdieu, Pierre. 1977. *Outline of a Theory of Practice*. Cambridge, U.K.: Cambridge University Press.

———. 1984. *Distinction*. Translated by R. Nice. Cambridge, Mass.: Harvard University Press.

———. 1990. *The Logic of Practice*. Translated by R. Nice. Stanford Calif.: Stanford University Press.

Bourdieu, Pierre, and Loïc J. D. Wacquant. 1992. *An Invitation to Reflexive Sociology*. Chicago: University of Chicago Press.

Boutenko, Irene A., and Kirill E. Razlogov. 1997. *Recent Social Trends in Russia 1960–1995*. Montreal: McGill-Queens University Press.

Brenner, M. Harvey. 1973. *Mental Illness and the Economy*. Cambridge, Mass.: Harvard University Press.

———. 1987. Economic Change, Alcohol Consumption and Disease Mortality in Nine Industrilized Countries. *Social Science and Medicine* 25:119–32.

Bridger, Sue. 1997. Rural Women and the Impact of Economic Change. Pp. 38–55 in *Post-Soviet Women: From the Baltic to Central Asia*, edited by M. Buckley. Cambridge, U.K.: Cambridge University Press.

Brodniak, Wlodzimierz Adam. 1996. Psychosocial Determinants of Nicotinism: Selected Findings. Paper presented at the European Society of Health and Medical Sociology meeting, August, Budapest, Hungary.

Brown, Halina Szejnawald, Robert Goble, and Henry K. Kirschner. 1995. Social and Environmental Factors in Lung Cancer Mortality in Post-War Poland. *Environmental Health Perspectives* 103:64–70.

Brown, Julie V., and Nina L. Rusinova. 1997. Russian Medical Care in the 1990s: A User's Perspective. *Social Science and Medicine* 45:1265–76.

Brym, Robert J. 1996. The Ethic of Self-Reliance and the Spirit of Capitalism in Russia. *International Sociology* 11:409–26.

Brzezinski, Zbigniew. 1989. *The Grand Failure: The Birth and Death of Communism in the Twentieth Century*. New York: Charles Scribner's Sons.

Buchmann, Marlis. 1989. *The Script of Life in Modern Society*. Chicago: University of Chicago Press.

Buckley, Mary, ed. 1997. *Post-Soviet Women: From the Baltic to Central Asia*. Cambridge, U.K.: Cambridge University Press.

Burawoy, Michael, and Pavel Krotov. 1992. The Soviet Transition from Socialism to Capitalism: Worker Control and Economic Bargaining in the Wood Industry. *American Sociological Review* 57:16–38.

Carlson, Elwood. 1989. Concentration of Rising Hungarian Mortality Among Manual Workers. *Sociology and Social Research* 73:119–27.

Carlson, Elwood, and Jitka Rychtaříková. 1996. Renewed Mortality Decline in the Czech Republic. Paper presented at the Sawyer-Mellon Conference on Increasing Adult Mortality in Eastern Europe, March, University of

Michigan, Ann Arbor, Michigan.

Carlson, Elwood, and Sergey Tsvetarsky. 1992. Concentration of Rising Bulgarian Mortality Among Manual Workers. *Sociology and Social Research* 76:81–4.

Cassileth, Barrie R., Vasily V. Vlassov, and Christopher C. Chapman. 1995. Health Care, Medical Practice, and Medical Ethics in Russia Today. *Journal of the American Medical Association* 273:1569–622.

Castells, Manuel. 1998. *End of Millennium*, vol. 3, *The Information Age: Economy, Society, and Culture*. Oxford, U.K.: Blackwell.

Centrul de Calcul si Statistica Sanitara [Central Health Statistics Office]. 1992. Consumul de Alcool si Tutun al Populatiei [Consumption of alcohol in the population]. Bucharest: Ministry of Health.

———. 1996. Anuar de statistica Sanitara 1995 [Annual health statistics 1995]. Bucharest: Ministry of Health.

Chamberlain, Lesley. 1982. *The Food and Cooking of Russia*. London: Penguin.

Chaney, David. 1996. *Lifestyles*. London: Routledge.

Cockerham, William C. 1996. *Sociology of Mental Disorder*. 4th ed. Upper Saddle River, N.J.: Prentice Hall.

———. 1997. The Social Determinants of the Decline of Life Expectancy in Russia and Eastern Europe: A Lifestyle Explanation. *Journal of Health and Social Behavior* 38:117–30.

———. 1998. *Medical Sociology*. 7th ed. Englewood Cliffs, N.J.: Prentice-Hall.

Cockerham, William C., Thomas Abel, and Günther Lüschen. 1993. Max Weber, Formal Rationality, and Health Lifestyles. *Sociological Quarterly* 34:413–25.

Cockerham, William C., Gerhard Kunz, and Guenther Lueschen. 1988. Social Stratification and Health Lifestyles in Two Systems of Health Care Delivery: A Comparison of America and West Germany. *Journal of Health and Social Behavior* 29:113–26.

Cockerham, William C., and Ferris J. Ritchey. 1997. *Dictionary of Medical Sociology*. Westport, Conn.: Greenwood Press.

Cockerham, William C., Alfred Rütten, and Thomas Abel. 1997. Conceptualizing Contemporary Health Lifestyles: Moving Beyond Weber. *Sociological Quarterly* 38:601–22.

Cockerham, William C., Yukio Yamori, and Hiroyuki Hattori. 1998. The Social Gradient in Life Expectancy: The Contrary Case of Japan and Okinawa. Paper presented at the American Sociological Association meetings, August, San Francisco, California.

Coleman, Fred. 1996. *The Decline and Fall of the Soviet Empire*. New York: St. Martin's Press.

Colton, Timothy J. 1995. *Moscow: Governing the Socialist Metropolis*. Cambridge, Mass.: Belknap Press of Harvard University.

Crawford, Robert. 1984. A Cultural Account of Health: Control, Release, and the Social Body. Pp. 60–103 in *Issues in the Political Economy of Health Care*, edited by J. McKinley. New York: Tavistock.

Crook, Stephen, Jan Pakulski, and Malcolm Waters. 1992. *Postmodernization: Change in Advanced Society*. London: Sage.

Csaszi, Lajos. 1990. Interpreting Inequalities in the Hungarian Health System. *Social Science and Medicine* 31:275–84.

Curtis, Sarah, Natasha Petukhova, and Ann Taket. 1995. Health Care Reforms in Russia: The Example of St. Petersburg. *Social Science and Medicine* 40:755–65.

Dahrendorf, Ralf. 1979. *Life Chances*. Chicago: University of Chicago Press.

Davies, Norman. 1984. *Heart of Europe: A Short History of Poland*. New York: Oxford University Press.

———. 1996. *Europe: A History*. New York: Oxford University Press.

Davis, Christopher M. 1989. The Soviet Health System: A National Health Service in a Socialist Society. Pp. 233–62 in *Success and Crisis in National Health Systems*, edited by M. Field. London: Routledge.

Davis, Christopher M., and Murray Feshbach. 1980. *Rising Infant Mortality in the U.S.S.R. in the 1970s*. Washington, D.C.: U.S. Bureau of the Census.

Deacon, Bob. 1984. Medical Care and Health Under State Socialism. *International Journal of Health Services* 14:453–82.

Dean, Kathryn. 1989. Self-Care Components of Lifestyles: The Importance of Gender, Attitudes, and the Social Situation. *Social Science and Medicine* 29:137–52.

Dennis, Mike. 1985. *German Democratic Republic*. London: Pinter.

Denzin, Norman K. 1991. *Images of Postmodern Society*. London: Sage.

d'Houtaud, A., and Mark G. Field. 1984. The Image of Health: Variations in Perception by Social Class. *Sociology of Health and Illness* 6:30–59.

Dogaru, Mircea, and Mihail Zahariade. 1996. *History of the Romanians: From the Origins to Modern Age*. Bucharest: Amco Press.

Domański, Henry. 1994. The Recomposition of Social Stratification in Poland. *Polish Sociological Review* 4:335–57.

Dumitrascu, D. L., S. Hopulele, and A. Baban. 1993. Cardiovascular Complaints Following the Uprising of December 1989 in Romania. *Medicine and War* 9:45–51.

Dwyer, Jeffrey W., Leslie L. Clarke, and Michael K. Miller. 1990. The Effect of Religious Concentration and Affiliation on County Cancer Mortality Rates. *Journal of Health and Social Behavior* 31:185–202.

Eberstadt, Nicholas. 1990. Health and Mortality in Eastern Europe, 1965–1985. *Communist Economies* 2:349–65.

———. 1994. Health and Mortality in Central and Eastern Europe: Retrospect and Prospect. Pp. 198-225 in *The Social Legacy of Communism*, edited by J. Millar and S. Wolchik. New York and Cambridge, U.K.: Woodrow Wilson Center Press and Cambridge University Press.

Emirbayer, Mustafa, and Ann Mische. 1998. What is Agency? *American Journal of Sociology* 103:962–1023.

Erdei, Ferenc. 1988. *Selected Writings*. Budapest: Akadémiai Kiadó.

Esping-Anderson, Gosta, ed. 1993. *Changing Classes: Stratification and Mobility in Post-Industrial Societies.* London: Sage.

Evans, Robert G. 1994. Introduction. Pp. 3-26 in *Why Are Some People Healthy and Others Not? The Determinants of Health of Populations,* edited by R. Evans, M. Barer, and T. Marmor. New York: Aldine de Gruyter.

Evans, Robert G., Morris L. Barer, and Theodore R. Marmor, eds. 1994. *Why Are Some People Healthy and Others Not? The Determinants of Health of Populations.* New York: Aldine de Gruyter.

Evans, Robert G., and G. L. Stoddard. 1994. Producing Health, Consuming Health Care. Pp. 2–64 in *Why Are Some People Healthy and Others Not? The Determinants of Health of Populations,* edited by R. Evans, M. Barer, and T. Marmor. New York: Aldine de Gruyter.

Feachem, R. 1994. Health Decline in Eastern Europe. *Nature* 367:313–14.

Featherstone, Mike. 1987. Lifestyle and Consumer Culture. *Theory, Culture and Society* 4:55–70.

———, ed. 1991. *Consumer Culture and Postmodernism.* London: Sage

Field, Mark G. 1967. *Soviet Socialized Medicine: An Introduction.* New York: Free Press.

———. 1991. The Hybrid Profession: Soviet Medicine. Pp. 43–62 in *Professions and the State,* edited by A. Jones. Philadelphia: Temple University Press.

———. 1993. The Physician in the Commonwealth of Independent States: The Difficult Passage from Bureaucrat to Professional. Pp. 162–83 in *The Changing Medical Profession,* edited by F. Hafferty and J. McKinlay. New York: Oxford University Press.

———. 1994. Postcommunist Medicine: Morbidity, Mortality, and the Deteriorating Health Situation. Pp. 178–95 in *The Social Legacy of Communism,* edited by J. Millar and S. Wollchik. New York and Cambridge, U.K.: Woodrow Wilson Center Press and Cambridge University Press.

———. 1995. The Health Crisis in the Former Soviet Union: A Report from the "Post-War" Zone. *Social Science and Medicine* 41:1469–78.

Figes, Orlando. 1996. *A People's Tragedy: A History of the Russian Revolution.* New York: Viking.

Forster, D. P., and Peter Józan. 1990. Health in Eastern Europe. *Lancet* 335:458–60.

Fulbrook, Mary. 1993. *A Concise History of Germany.* Updated edition. Cambridge, U.K.: Cambridge University Press.

Garrett, Laurie. 1997. Former Soviet Union: Health Disaster in the Making. *Birmingham News* (30 November): 9A

Geisser, Rainer. 1996. *Die Sozialstruktur Deutschlands.* [The social structure of Germany]. Opladen: Westdeutscher Verlag.

Giddens, Anthony. 1984. *The Constitution of Society: Outline of the Theory of Structration.* Cambridge: Polity Press.

———. 1991. *Modernity and Self-Identity.* Stanford: Stanford University Press.

Ginter, Emil. 1997. The Influence of Some Factors on the Non-Homogeneity in Adult Male Life Expectancy in the Slovak Republic. *Central European Journal of Public Health* 5:133–5.

Ginter, Emil, Milan Tatara, and Tatjana Sipekiová. 1995. Nehomogenita strednej dĺžky žiuota na Slovensku [Non-homogeneity of life expectancy in Slovakia]. *Bratislavske Lekarske Listy* 6:301–6.

Glenny, Misha. 1993. *The Rebirth of History: Eastern Europe in a Time of Democracy.* New edition. London: Penguin.

Godek, Lisa. 1995. The Gender Gap in Ukrainian Mortality. Paper presented at the Sawyer-Mellon Conference on Increasing Adult Mortality in Eastern Europe, December, University of Michigan, Ann Arbor, Michigan.

Goldman, Marshall I. 1996. *Lost Opportunity: What Has Made Economic Reform in Russia So Difficult?* New York: Norton.

Goldstein, Michael S. 1992. *The Health Movement: Promoting Fitness in America.* New York: Twayne.

Gorbachev, Mikhail. 1996. *Memoirs.* Translated by G. Peronansky and T. Varsavsley. New York: Doubleday.

Gordon, Michael R. 1997. On the Road to Capitalism, Tax Breakdown for Russia. *New York Times* (19 February): A1, A5.

Graham, Lawrence S. 1982. *Romania: A Developing Socialist State.* Boulder, Colo.: Westview Press.

Gray, Francine du Plessix. 1990. *Soviet Women.* New York: Doubleday.

Gzyl, J. 1997. Assessment of Polish Population Exposure to Lead and Cadmium with Special Emphasis to the Katowice Province on the Basis of Metal Concentrations in Environmental Compartments. *Central European Journal of Public Health* 5:93–6.

Hafferty, Frederic W., and Donald W. Light. 1995. Professional Dynamics and the Changing Nature of Medical Work. *Journal of Health and Social Behavior* Extra Issue: 132–53.

Harvey, David. 1989. *The Condition of Postmodernity.* Oxford, U.K.: Blackwell.

Haub, Carl. 1994. Population Change in the Former Soviet Republics. *Population Bulletin*, vol. 49. Washington, D.C.: Population Reference Bureau.

Häussler, B., Elke Hempel, and P. Reschke. 1995. Die Entwicklung von Lebenserwartung und Sterblichkeit in Ostdeutschland nach der Wende (1989–1992) [Life expectancy and mortality in East Germany after the fall of the Berlin Wall (1989–1992)] *Gesundheitswesen* 7:365–72.

Heinemann, L., W. Barth, and H. Hoffmeister. 1995. Trend of Cardiovascular Risk Factors in the East German Population. *Journal of Clinical Epidemiology* 48:787–95.

Heinemann, L., R. Dinkel, and E. Görtler. 1996. Life Expectancy in Germany: Possible Reasons for the Increasing Gap Between East and West Germany. *Reviews on Environmental Health* 11:15–26.

Heitlinger, Alena. 1993. The Medical Profession in Czechoslovakia: Legacies of State Socialism, Prospects for the Capitalist Future. Pp. 172–83 in *The Changing Medical Profession*, edited by F. Hafferty and J. McKinley. New York: Oxford University Press.

Helmert, Uwe, Andreas Mielck, and Elvira Classen. 1992. Social Inequities in Cardiovascular Disease Risk Factors in East and West Germany. *Social*

Science and Medicine 35:1283–92.

Hertrich, Véronique, and France Meslé. 1997. Mortality by Cause in Baltic Countries Since 1970: A Method for Reconstructing Time Series. Paper presented at the Demographic Development in the Baltic Countries International Symposium, April, Tallin, Estonia.

Hertzman, Clyde. 1995. *Environment and Health in Central and Eastern Europe*. Washington, D.C.: World Bank.

Hertzman, Clyde, J. Frank, and Robert G. Evans. 1994. Heterogeneities in Health Status and the Determinants of Population Health. Pp. 67–92 in *Why Are Some People Healthy and Others Not? The Determinants of Health of Populations*, edited by R. Evans, M. Barer, and T. Marmor. New York: Aldine de Gruyter.

Herzlich, Claudine, and Janine Pierret. 1987. *Illness and Self in Society*. Translated by E. Forster. Baltimore: Johns Hopkins University Press.

Hitzler, Ronald, and Elmar Koenen. 1994. Kehren die Individuen zurück? Zwei divergente Antworten auf eine institutionentheoretische Frage [Are individuals returning? Two divergent answers to questions of institutional theory]. Pp. 447–65 in *Riskante Freiheiten*, edited by U. Beck and E. Beck-Gernsheim. Frankfurt am Main: Suhrkamp.

Holmes, Leslie. 1997. *Post-Communism: Introduction*. Durham, N.C.: Duke University Press.

Hraba, Joseph, Frederick O. Lorenz, Gang Lee, and Zdenka Pechacova. 1996. Gender and Well-Being in the Czech Republic. *Sex Roles: A Journal of Research* 34:517–34.

Hradil, Stefan. 1987. *Sozialstrukturanalyse in einer fortgeschrittenen Gesellschaft* [Social structural analysis in an advanced society]. Leverkusen: Leske and Budrich.

Hungarian Central Statistical Office. 1995. Preliminary Report on the Health Behavior Survey–94. Budapest.

———. 1996. Main Features of the Hungarian Demographic Situation in the Early Nineties. Budapest.

———. 1997. *Demographic Yearbook 1995*. Budapest.

Hungarian Ministry of Welfare. 1995. Program of Health Services Modernization: Supplements. Budapest.

Hurt, Richard D. 1995. Smoking in Russia: What Do Stalin and Western Tobacco Companies Have in Common? *Mayo Clinic Proceedings* 70:1007–11.

Illsley, R., and D. Baker. 1991. Contextual Variations in the Meaning of Health Inequality. *Social Science and Medicine* 32:359–65.

Institute of Health Information and Statistics of the Czeck Republic. 1995. HIS CR 93 Sample Survey of the Health Status of the Czech Population. Prague.

———. 1997. Health Care and Health Services in the Czech Republic 1996. Prague.

Interstate Statistical Committee of the Commonwealth of Independent States. 1995. *Demographic Yearbook 1994*. Moscow.

Jahrbuch der Bundesrepublik [Yearbook of the Federal Republic of Germany]. 1996. Munich: Beck.

Jameson, Frederic. 1991. *Postmodernism or, The Cultural Logic of Late Capitalism*. Durham, N.C.: Duke Univesity Press.

Janečková, Hana, and Helena Hniličová. 1992. The Health Status of the Czechoslovak Population. Its Social and Ecological Determinants. *International Journal of Health Sciences* 3:143–56.

Jarausch, Konrad H. 1994. *The Rush to German Unity*. New York: Oxford University Press.

Jaspers, Karl. 1988. *On Max Weber*. Edited by J. Dreijmans. New York: Paragon House.

Jenkins, Richard. 1992. *Pierre Bourdieu*. London: Routledge.

Józan, Peter. 1989. Some Features of Mortality in Postwar Hungary: The Third Epidemiological Transition. *Cahiers de Sociologie Démographie Médicales* 29:21–42.

———. 1996a. Health Crisis East of the Elbe: A Consequence of Death-Ended Modernization. Paper presented at the Sawyer-Mellon Conference on Increasing Adult Mortality in Eastern Europe, March, University of Michigan, Ann Arbor, Michigan.

———. 1996b. Main Features of the Hungarian Demographic Situation in the Early Nineties. Pp. 9–20 in *Annual Report 1996*, edited by A. Czeizel. Budapest: National Institute for Health Promotion.

Kaasik, Taie, Lars-Gunnar Hörte, and Ragnar Andersson. 1996. *Injury in Estonia: An Estonian-Swedish Comparative Study*. Sundbyberg, Sweden: Karolinska Institute.

Kalberg, Stephen. 1994. *Max Weber's Comparative Historical Sociology*. Chicago: University of Chicago Press.

Kaplan, Robert D. 1993. *Balkan Ghosts: A Journey Through History*. London: Papermac.

Keep, John. 1995. *Last of the Empires: A History of the Soviet Union 1945–1991*. Oxford, U.K.: Oxford University Press.

Kerekovska, A., and Nevyana Feschieva. 1995. Health Behavior—Socio-Demographic Determinants, Varna–1995. Unpublished manuscript. Varna, Bulgaria: Medical University of Varna, Department of Social Medicine.

Kirschbaum, Stanislav J. 1995. *A History of Slovakia: The Struggle for Survival*. New York: St. Martin's Griffin.

Kliment, V., R. Kubínová, H. Kazmarová, B. Havlík, P. Šišma, J. Ruprich, M. Černá, and M. Kodl. 1997. System of Monitoring the Environmental Impact on Population Health of the Czech Republic. *Central European Journal of Public Health* 5(3):107–16.

Knaus, William A. 1981. *Inside Russian Medicine*. Boston: Beacon Press.

Knox, Richard. 1993. *Germany's Health System*. Washington, D.C.: Faulkner and Gray.

Kochetov, Aleksei. 1993. Istoki "novoi" sotdial'noi struktury [Beginning of the new social structure]. *Svobodnaia mysl* 9:68.

Kohn, Melvin L., and Kazimierz Slomczyński. 1990. *Social Structure and Self-*

Direction: A Comparative Analysis of the United States and Poland. Oxford, U.K.: Blackwell.

Kohn, Melvin L., Kazimierz M. Slomczyński, Krystyna Jamicka, Valeri Khmelko, Bogdan W. Mach, Vladimir Paniotto, Wojciech Zaborowski, Roberto Gutierrez, and Cory Heyman. 1997. Social Structure and Personality Under Conditions of Radical Social Change: A Comparative Analysis of Poland and Ukraine. *American Sociological Review* 62:614–38.

Kolosi, Tamás, and Ivan Szelényi. 1993. Social Change and Research on Social Structure in Hungary. Pp. 141–164 in *Sociology in Europe: In Search of Identity*, edited by B. Nedelmann and P. Sztompka. Berlin: Aldine de Gruyter.

Krumins, Juris. 1997. Health and Mortality During a Transition to a Market Economy: Case of Latvia. Paper presented at the Demographic Development in the Baltic Countries International Symposium, April, Tallin, Estonia.

Kubik, Antonin, D. Maxwell Parkin, Ivan Plesko, Witold Zatonski, Eva Kramarova, Matthias Möhner, Hans P. Friedl, Lajos Juhasz, Christo G. Tzvetansky, and Jindra Reissigova. 1995. Patterns of Cigarette Sales and Lung Cancer Mortality in Some Central and Eastern European Countries, 1960–1989. *Cancer* 75:2452–560.

Kučera, Milan, and Zdeněk Pavlík. 1995. Czech and Slovak Demography. Pp. 15–39 in *The End of Czechoslovakia*, edited by J. Musil. Budapest: Central European Univesity Press.

Kuchuk, Alexander A. 1994. Health Problems of the Population in Different Regions of the Ukraine. *Toxicology Letters* 72:213–17.

Kulin, Howard E., and Niels E. Skakkeback. 1995. Environmental Effects on Human Reproduction: The Basis for New Efforts in Eastern Europe. *Social Science and Medicine* 41:1479–86.

Kwasniewicz, Wladyslaw. 1993. Between Universal and Native: The Case of Polish Sociology. Pp. 165–88 in *Sociology in Europe: In Search of Identity*, edited by B. Nedelmann and P. Sztompka. Berlin: Aldine de Gruyter.

Laqueur, Walter. 1994. *The Dream That Failed: Reflections on the Soviet Union.* New York: Oxford University Press.

Lash, Scott. 1990. *Sociology of Postmodernism.* London: Routledge.

Lassey, Marie L., William R. Lassey, and Martin J. Jinks, eds. 1997. *Health Care Systems Around the World.* Upper Saddle River, N.J.: Prentice Hall.

Lemert, Charles, ed. 1993. *Social Theory: The Multicultural and Classic Readings.* Boulder, Colo.: Westview Press.

Leon, David A., and Vladimir M. Shkolnikov. 1998. Social Stress and the Russian Mortality Crisis. *Journal of the American Medical Association* 279:790–91.

Leon, David A., Laurent Chenet, Vladmir M. Shkolnikov, Sergei Zakharov, Judith Shapiro, Galina Rakhmanova, Sergei Vassin, and Martin McKee. 1997. Huge Variation in Russian Mortality Rates 1984–94: Artefact, Alcohol, or What? *Lancet* 350:383–7.

Levi, F., C. La Vecchia, F. Lucchini, and E. Negri. 1995. Cancer Mortality in Europe, 1990–92. *European Journal of Cancer Prevention* 4:389–417.

Lewis, Flora. 1987. *Europe: A Tapestry of Nations*. New York: Simon and Schuster.

Light, Donald W. 1986. Introduction: State, Profession, and Political Values. Pp. 1–23 in *Political Values and Health Care: The German Experience*, edited by D. Light and A. Schuller. Cambridge, Mass.: MIT Press.

———. 1992. Russia: Perestroika for Health Care? *Lancet* 339:326.

Light, Donald W., and Alexander Schuller, eds. 1986. *Political Values and Health Care: The German Experience*. Cambridge, Mass.: MIT Press.

Lovenduski, Joni, and Jean Woodall. 1987. *Politics and Society in Eastern Europe*. Bloomington, Ind.: Indiana University Press.

Löwith, Karl. 1982. *Max Weber and Karl Marx*. Edited by T. Bottomore and W. Outhwaite. London: Allen and Unwin.

Lukacs, John. 1988. *Budapest 1900: A Historical Portrait of a City and Its Culture*. New York: Grove Press.

Lüschen, Günther, and Peter Apelt. 1992. Health Situation and Social Stratification in East and West Germany. Paper presented at the British Sociological Association Medical Sociology Group meeting, September, Edinburgh, Scotland.

Lüschen, Günther, Peter Apelt, and Gerhard Kunz. 1993. Systems in Transition: Health Conduct. Health Care and Social Stratification in East and West Germany. Paper presented at the Midwest Sociological Society meeting, April, Chicago, Illinois.

Lüschen, Günther, William Cockerham, Jouke van der Zee, Fred Stevens, Jos Diederiks, Manuel Garcia Ferrando, Alphonse d'Houtaud, Ruud Peeters, Thomas Abel, and Steffen Niemann. 1995. *Health Systems in the European Union: Diversity, Convergence, and Integration*. Munich: Oldenbourg.

Lüschen, Günther, Olga Geling, Christian Janssen, Gerhard Kunz, and Olaf von dem Knesebeck. 1997. After Unification: Gender and Subjective Health Status in East and West Germany. *Social Science and Medicine* 44:1313–23.

Lüschen, Günther, Steffen Niemann, and Peter Apelt. 1997. The Integration of Two Health Systems: Social Stratification, Work, and Health in East and West Germany. *Social Science and Medicine* 44:833–99.

Mackenbach, J. P., C. W. Looman, A. E. Kunst, J. D. Habbema, and P. J. van de Maas. 1988. Post-1950 Mortality Trends and Medical Care: Gains in Life Expectancy Due to Declines in Mortality From Conditions Amenable to Medical Intervention in The Netherlands. *Social Science and Medicine* 27:889–94.

Maffesoli, Michel. 1996. *The Time of Tribes: The Decline of Individualism in Mass Society*. London: Sage.

Makara, Peter. 1994. Policy Implications of Differential Health Status in East and West Europe: The Case of Hungary. *Social Science and Medicine* 39:1295–1302.

Makowiec-Dabrowska, T. 1995. Czy ciezka praca fizyczna jest czynnikiem ryzyka choroby niedokrwiennej serca? [Is heavy work a risk factor in heart disease?]. *Medycyna Pracy* 46:263–74.

Marel, M., L. Melinova, B. Stastny, Z. Skacel, R. Marelova, M. Jechova, and J. Krenarova. 1996. Vyvoj epidemiologickych ukazatelu plicni rakoviny v Ceske republice v letech 1970–1990 [Trends in epidemiological indicators of lung cancer in the Czech Republic 1970–1990]. *Časopis Lékařu Českých* 135:487–92.

Mark, L., A. Kondacs, and V. Hanyecz. 1997. Kardiovaskulare Riskiofaktoren: Vergleich einer ungarischen Gemeinde mit Deutschland [Cardiovascular risk factors: Comparison of a Hungarian community with Germany]. *Weiner Klinische Wochenschrift* 109:683–87.

Marmot, Michael G. 1996. Socioeconomic Factors in Cardiovascular Disease. *Journal of Hypertension* 14:5201–5.

Marmot, Michael G., J. Shipley, and Geoffrey Rose. 1984. Inequalities in Death-Specific Explanations of a General Pattern. *Lancet* 83:1003–6.

Marmot, Michael G., G. D. Smith, S. Stansfeld, C. Patel, F. North, J. Head, I. White, E. Brunner, and A. Feeney. 1991. Health Inequalities Among British Civil Servants: The Whitehall II Study. *Lancet* 337:1387–93.

Marrée, Jörgen, and Peter P. Groenewegen. 1997. *Back to Bismarck: Eastern European Health Care System in Transition*. Aldershot, U.K.: Avebury.

Marshall, T. H. 1964. *Class, Citizenship, and Social Development*. Chicago: University of Chicago Press.

Marx, Karl, and Friedrich Engels. [1846] 1973. *The German Ideology*. Moscow: Progress Publishers.

Massaro, Thomas A., Jiri Nemec, and Ivan Kalman. 1994. Health System Reform in the Czech Republic: Policy Lessons from the Initial Experience of the General Health Insurance Company. *Journal of the American Medical Association* 271:1870–74.

Massie, Robert K. 1995. *The Romanovs: The Final Chapter.* New York: Ballantine.

McDaniel, Tim. 1996. *The Agony of the Russian Idea*. Princeton, N.J.: Princeton University Press.

McKeehan, Irina V. 1995. Planning of National Primary Health Care and Prevention Programs: The First Health Insurance Law of Russia, 1992–1993. Pp. 174–97 in *Global Perspecitves on Health Care*, edited by E. Gallagher and J. Subedi. Englewood Cliffs, N.J: Prentice Hall.

Meslé, France, and Vladimir M. Shkolnikov. 1995. La mortalité en Russie: une crise sanitaire en deux temps [Mortality in Russia: A health crisis in two periods]. *Revue d'études comparatives Est-Ouest* 4:9–24.

Meslé, France, Vladimir M. Shkolnikov, Véronique Hertrich, and Jacques Vallin. 1996. *Tendances récentes de la mortalité par cause en Russie 1965–1994* [Recent trends in mortality by cause in Russia 1965–1994]. Paris and Moscow: Institut national d'etudes démographiques (Paris) and Centre de démographie et d'écologie humaine (Moscow).

Meslé, France, Vladimir M. Shkolnikov, and Jacques Vallin. 1992. Mortality by Cause in the U.S.S.R. in 1970–1987: The Reconstruction of Time Series.

European Journal of Population 8:281–308.

Meštrovic, Stjepan G. 1991. *The Coming Fin De Siècle*. London: Routledge.

———. 1992. *Durkheim and Postmodern Culture*. London: Routledge.

Mezentseva, Elena, and Natalia Rimachevskaya. 1990. The Soviet Country Profile: Health of the U.S.S.R. Population in the '70s and '80s—An Approach to a Comprehensive Analysis. *Social Science and Medicine* 31:867–77.

———. 1992. The Health of the Populations in the Republics of the Former Soviet Union: An Analysis of the Situation in the 1970s and 1980s. *International Journal of the Health Sciences* 3:127–42.

Mihăilă, Valentina, Dan Enăchescu, and Maria Bădulescu. 1996. A Short Form of the 36 (SF-36) Health Questionnaire: Normative Data for the Romanian Population. Bucharest: Institute of Hygiene, Public Health, Health Services and Management.

Millard, Frances L. 1984. Health Care in Poland: From Crisis to Crisis. *International Journal of Health Services* 12:497–515.

Minev, Duchomir, Bogdana Dermendjieva, and Natasha Mileva. 1990. The Bulgarian Country Profile: The Dynamics of Some Inequalities in Health. *Social Science and Medicine* 31:837–46.

Mirowsky, John, and Catherine E. Ross. 1989. *Social Causes of Psychological Distress*. New York: Aldine de Gruyter.

Mommsen, Wolfgang J. 1989. *The Political and Social Theory of Max Weber*. Cambridge, U.K.: Polity Press.

Münch, Richard. 1988. *Understanding Modernity*. London: Routledge.

———. 1993. The Contributions of German Social Theory to European Sociology. Pp. 45–66 in *Sociology in Europe*, edited by B. Nedelmann and P. Sztompka. Berlin: Aldine de Gruyter.

Muresan, Cornelia. 1996. The Decrease of Life-Expectancy at Birth and the Economism of the Sanitary Reform. Paper presented at the European Society of Health and Medical Sociology, September, Budapest, Hungary.

Musil, Jiří. 1995. Czech and Slovak Society. Pp. 77-94 in *The End of Czechoslovakia*, edited by J. Musil. Budapest: Central European University Press.

Myles, John F. 1984. *Old Age in the Welfare State*. Boston: Little, Brown.

Nagorski, Andrew. 1993. *The Birth of Freedom: Shaping Lives and Societies in the New Eastern Europe*. New York: Simon and Schuster.

Naseleniye SSR [Population of the U.S.S.R.]. 1962. Moscow: Finnansy i Statistika.

National Center of Health Informatics. 1995. Public Health Statistics Annual, Bulgaria 1994. Sofia: Ministry of Health.

National Center for Health System Management. 1996. Health Care System in Transition (HIT) Profile Poland. Warsaw: Ministry of Health and Social Welfare.

———. 1997. *Health Care in Numbers*. Warsaw: Ministry of Health and Social Welfare.

Navarro, Vicente. 1986. *Crisis, Health, and Medicine: A Social Critique.* New York: Tavistock.

Nemtsov, Alexander V., and Vladimir M. Shkolnikov. 1994. Jit' ili pit'? [To live or to drink?]. *Izvestiya* (19 July):22–3.

Niehoff, J. U., F. Schneider, and E. Wetzstein. 1992. Reflections on the Health Policy of the Former German Democratic Republic. *International Journal of Health Services* 3:205–13.

Notzon, Francis C., Yuri M. Komarov, Sergei P. Ermakov, Christopher T. Sempos, James S. Marks, and Elena V. Sempos. 1998. Letter from Russia: Causes for Declining Life Expectancy in Russia. *Journal of the American Medical Association* 279:793–800.

Okólski, Marek. 1993. East-West Mortality Differentials. *European Population,* vol. 2. Edited by A. Blum and J. Rallu. London: John Libbey.

Opp, Karl-Dieter. 1991. Zu den Ursachen einer Spontanen Revolution [The causes of a spontaneous revolution]. *Kölner Zeitschrift für Soziologie und Sozialpsychologie* 43:302–21.

Opp, Karl-Dieter, and Christiane Gern. 1993. Dissident Groups, Personal Networks, and Spontaneous Cooperation: The East German Revolution of 1989. *American Sociological Review* 8:659–80.

Organization for Economic Cooperation and Development (OECD). 1996. *Poland 1997.* Paris: Organization for Economic Co-Operation and Development.

Orosz, Eva. 1990. The Hungarian Country Profile: Inequalities in Health and Health Care in Hungary. *Social Science and Medicine* 31:847–57.

———. 1996. Main Challenges for Health Policy in a Period of Socio-Economic Transformation in Hungary. Paper presented at the European Society of Health and Medical Society meeting, August, Budapest, Hungary.

Ostrowska, Antonina. 1993. From Totalitarianism to Pluralism in Poland. *European Journal of Public Health* 3:43–7.

———. 1996. The Development of Medical Sociology in Eastern Europe, 1965–1990. *European Journal of Public Health* 6:100–4.

———. 1997. Prozdrowotne style zycia [Healthy lifestyles]. Unpublished manuscript. Warsaw, Polish Academy of Sciences, Institute of Philosophy and Sociology.

Palosuo, Hannele. 1997. Alienation, Lifestyle, and Health in Helsinki and Moscow. Paper presented at the Seminar on Lifestyle and Health, May, University of Helsinki, Helsinki, Finland.

Palosuo, Hannele, Antti Uutele, Irina Zhuravleva, and Nina Lakomova. 1998. Social Patterning of Ill Health in Helsinki and Moscow: Results from a Comparative Survey in 1991. *Social Science and Medicine* 46:1121–36.

Palosuo, Hannele, Irina Zhuravleva, Antti Uutela, Nina Lakomova, and Lyudmila Shilova. 1995. *Perceived Health, Health-Related Habits and Attitudes in Helsinki and Moscow: A Comparative Study of Adult Population in 1991.* Helsinki, Finland: National Public Health Institute.

Pearlin, Leonard I. 1989. The Sociological Study of Stress. *Journal of Health and Social Behavior* 30:241–56.

Peters, A., I. F. Goldstein, U. Beyer, K. Franke, J. Heinrich, D. W. dockery, J. D. Spengler, and H. E. Wichmann. 1996. Acute Health Effects of Exposure to High Levels of Air Pollution in Eastern Europe. *American Journal of Epidemiology* 144:570–81.

Peto, Richard, Alan D. Lopez, Jillian Boreham, Micheal Thun, and Clark Heath. 1992. Mortality from Tobacco in Developed Countries: Indirect Estimation from National Vital Statistics. *Lancet* 339:1268–78.

Pipes, Richard. 1995. *Russia Under the Old Regime*. 2d ed. London: Penguin.

Polednak, Melvin. 1989. *Racial and Ethnic Differences in Disease*. New York: Oxford University Press.

Ponarin, E. 1996. Adult Mortality and Alcohol Consumption in Russia. Paper presented at the Sawyer-Mellon Conference on Increasing Adult Mortality in Eastern Europe, March, University of Michigan, Ann Arbor, Michigan.

Popkin, Barry M., Namvar Zohoori, and Alexander Baturin. 1996. The Nutritional Status of the Elderly in Russia, 1992 through 1994. *American Journal of Public Health* 86:355–60.

Popova, Stoyanka, and Nevyana Feschieva. 1995. The State of Primary Medical Care in Bulgaria. *Journal of Public Health Medicine* 17:6-10.

Potrykowska, Alina. 1995. The Effects of Environmental Pollution for Population in Poland. Pp. 307–24 in *Population-Environment-Development Interactions*, edited by J. Clarke and L. Tabah. Paris: CICRED.

Prûcha, Václav. 1995. Economic Development and Relations, 1918–89. Pp. 40–76 in *The End of Czechoslovakia*, edited by J. Musil. Budapest: Central European University Press.

Pryce-Jones, David. 1995. *The Strange Death of the Soviet Empire*. New York: Metropolitan Books.

Radzinsky, Edvard. 1992. *The Last Tsar: The Life and Death of Nicholas II*. Translated by M. Schwartz. New York: Doubleday.

Raffel, M. W., and N. K. Raffel. 1992. Czechoslovakia's Changing Health Care System. *Public Health Reports* 6:636–43.

Remennick, Larissa I., and Ronny A. Shtarkshall. 1997. Technology Versus Responsibility: Immigrant Physicians from the Former Soviet Union Reflect on Israeli Health Care. *Journal of Health and Social Behavior* 38:191–202.

Remnick, David. 1993. *Lenin's Tomb: The Last Days of the Soviet Empire*. New York: Random House.

———. 1997. *Resurrection: The Struggle for a New Russia*. New York: Random House.

Richie, Alexandra. 1998. *Faust's Metropolis: A History of Berlin*. New York: Carroll and Graf.

Rigby, T. H. 1990. *The Changing Soviet System: Monoorganizational Socialism from its Origins to Gorbachev's Restructuring*. Brookfield, U.K.: Edward Elgar.

Rimachevskaya, Natalia. 1993. The Individual's Health Is the Health of Society.

Sociological Research 32:22–34.

Ritzer, George. 1997. *Postmodern Social Theory*. New York: McGraw-Hill.

Roemer, Milton I. 1994. Recent Health System Development in Poland and Hungary. *Journal of Community Health* 19:153–62.

Roosevelt, Priscilla. 1995. *Life on the Russian Country Estate*. New Haven, Conn.: Yale University.

Rose, Cheryl D., and Arthur D. Bloom. 1994. Human Health and the Environment in Eastern Europe. *Environmental Health Perspectives* 102:696–8.

Rosenberg, Tina. 1995. *The Haunted Land: Facing Europe's Ghosts After Communism*. New York: Vintage.

Ross, Catherine E., and Chloe E. Bird. 1994. Sex Stratification and Health Lifestyle: Consequences for Men's and Women's Perceived Health. *Journal of Health and Social Behavior* 23:199–31.

Roth, Guenther. 1987. Rationalization in Max Weber's Developmental History. Pp. 75–91 in *Max Weber, Rationality and Modernism*, edited by S. Whimster and S. Lash. London: Allen & Unwin.

Rowland, Diane, and Alexandre V. Telyukov. 1991. Soviet Health Care from Two Perspectives. *Health Affairs* 10:71–86.

Roxburgh, Angus. 1992. *The Second Russian Revolution*. New York: Pharos.

Rozenfeld, Boris A. 1996. The Crisis of Russian Health Care and Attempts at Reform. Pp. 163–73 in *Russia's Demographic Crisis*, edited by J. DaVanzo. Santa Monica, Calif.: Rand Center for Russian and Eurasian Studies.

Rush, David, and Kathleen Welch. 1996. The First Year of Hyperinflation in the Former Soviet Union: Nutritional Deprivation Among Elderly Pensioners, 1992. *American Journal of Public Health* 86:361–7.

Ruzicka, Lado T., and Alan D. Lopez. 1990. The Use of Cause-of-Death Statistics for Health Situation Assessment: National and International Experiences. *World Health Statistics Quarterly* 43:249–58.

Ryan, Michael. 1993. Russian Report: Personalia and the Current Health Crisis. *British Medical Journal* 306:909–11.

———. 1995. Alcoholism and Rising Mortality in the Russian Federation. *British Medical Journal* 310:646–8.

Rychtaříková, Jitka. 1996. Will the Czech Republic Escape the Eastern European Crisis? Paper presented at the Sawyer-Mellon Conference on Increasing Adult Mortality in Eastern Europe, March, University of Michigan, Ann Arbor, Michigan.

Schieber, G. J., J. P. Poullier, and L. M. Greenwald. 1994. Data Watch. *Health Affairs* 13:100–12.

Schmemann, Serge. 1997. *Echoes of a Native Land: Two Centuries of a Russian Village*. New York: Knopf.

Seidman, Steven, ed. 1994. *The Postmodern Turn: New Perspectives on Social Theory*. Cambridge, U.K.: Cambridge University Press.

Seidman, Steven, and David G. Wagner, eds. 1992. *Postmodernism and Social*

Theory. Cambridge, Mass.: Blackwell.

Sekula, Wlodzimierz, Katarina Babinska, and Stefka Petrova. 1997. Nutrition Policies in Central and Eastern Europe. *Nutrition Review* 55:S58–S73.

Sewell, William H., Jr. 1992. A Theory of Structure: Duality, Agency, and Transformation. *American Journal of Sociology* 98:1–29.

Shapiro, Judith. 1995. The Russian Mortality Crisis and Its Causes. Pp. 149–78 in *Russian Economic Reform at Risk*, edited by A. Åslund. London: Pinter.

Sheahan, Michelle D. 1995. Prevention in Poland: Health Care System Reform. *Public Health Reports* 110:289–95.

Sheiman, Igor. 1994. Forming the System of Health Insurance in the Russian Federation. *Social Science and Medicine*, 39:1425–32.

Shilling, Chris. 1993. *The Body and Social Theory*. London: Sage.

Shkolnikov, Vladimir M. 1995. Recent Trends in Russian Mortality: 1993–1994. Paper presented at the USAID Conference, October, Moscow.

———. 1996. The Russian Health Crisis of the 1990s in Mortality Dimensions. Paper presented at the Common Security Forum Policy meeting, September, Stockholm.

———. 1997. Mortality and Life Expectancy. Pp. 113-34 in *Naseleniye Rossii 1996* [Population of Russia 1996], edited by A. Visherevskiy. Moscow: Center for Demography and Human Ecology.

Shkolnikov, Vladimir M., Sergey Adamets, and Alexander Deev. 1996. Mortality Differentials in the Context of General Mortality Reversal in Russia: The Educational Status. Paper presented at the Sawyer-Mellon Conference on Increasing Adult Mortality in Eastern Europe, March, University of Michigan, Ann Arbor, Michigan.

Shkolnikov, Vladimir M., and France Meslé. 1996. The Russian Epidemiological Crisis as Mirrored by Mortality Patterns. Pp. 113–62 in *Russia's Demographic Crisis*, edited by J. DaVanzo. Santa Monica, Calif.: RAND.

Shkolnikov, Vladimir M., France Meslé, and Jacques Vallin. 1996a. Health Crisis in Russia I. Recent Trends in Life Expectancy and Causes of Death from 1970 to 1993. *Population: An English Selection* 8:123–54.

———. 1996b. Health Crisis in Russia II. Changes in Causes of Death: A Comparison with France, England, and Wales (1970 to 1993). *Population: An English Selection* 8:155–90.

Shkolnikov, Vladimir, and Alexander Nemtsov. 1994. The Anti-Alcohol Campaign and Variations in Russian Mortality. Paper presented at the Workshop on Mortality and Adult Health Priorities in the New Independent States, November, Washington, D.C.

Sidel, Victor W., and Ruth Sidel. 1983. *A Healthy State: An International Perspective on the Crisis in United States Medical Care*. Rev. ed. New York: Pantheon.

Siegrist, Johannes. 1996. High Cost–Low Gain Conditions at Work as a Determinant of Cardiovascular Disease Morbidity and Mortality. Pp. 169–85 in *East-West Differences in Life Expectancy: Environmental and*

Nonenvironmental Determinants. Dordrecht, The Netherlands: Kulwer.

Sigerist, Henry E. 1947. *Medicine and Health in the Soviet Union.* New York: Citadel Press.

Skidelsky, Robert. 1995. *The Road from Serfdom: The Economic and Political Consequences of the End of Communism.* New York: Allen Lane.

Škodová, Z., R. Píša, L. Poledne, Z. Berka, Z. Cícha, R. Emrová, M. Hoke, J. Pikhartova, P. Vojtíšek, D. Grafnetter, E. Wiesner, K. Hardlíčková, A. Havlíková, M. Bobák, J. Volícek, M. Paclt, and V. Lánská. 1997. Pokles úmrtnosti na kardiovaskulární onemocěně ní v České republice v obdabí 1984–1993 a jeho možné príčiny [Decline of the cardiovascular mortality rate in the Czech Republic in 1984–1993 and its possible causes]. *Casopis Lékařů Ceskych* 136:373–79. (In Czech.)

Slomczyński, Kazimierz M. 1997. Systemic Formation and the Salience of Class Structure in East Central Europe. *East European Politics and Societies* 11:155–89.

Slomczyński, Kazimierz M., and Tadeusz K. Krauze, eds. 1986. *Social Stratification in Poland.* Armonk, N.Y.: Sharpe.

Slomczyński, Kazimierz M., and Goldie Shabad. 1997. Systematic Transformation and the Salience of Class Structure in East Central Europe. *East European Politics and Societies* 11:155–89.

Smart, Barry. 1992. *Modern Conditions, Postmodern Controversies.* London: Routledge.

———.1993. *Postmodernity.* London: Routledge.

Smelser, Neil J. 1988. Social Structure. Pp. 103–29 in *Handbook of Sociology,* edited by N. Smelser. Newbury Park, Calif.: Sage.

———. 1997. *Problematics of Sociology.* Berkeley: University of California Press.

Smith, Hendrick. 1990. *The New Russians.* New York: Random House.

Sokolowska, M., and B. Moskalewicz. 1987. Health Sector Structures: The Case of Poland. *Social Science and Medicine* 24:763–75.

Specter, Michael. 1995. Russia's Declining Health: Rising Illness, Shorter Lives. *New York Times* (19 February): 1, 4.

———. 1996. Ten Years Later, Through Fear, Chernobyl Still Kills in Belarus. *New York Times* (31 March): 1, 4.

———. 1997a. Needing Taxes, Yeltsin Takes on a Religion of the Russians: Vodka. *New York Times* (21 January): A1, A3.

———. 1997b. Onrush of AIDS Is Driving an Infirm Russia to Its Knees. *New York Times* (10 May): 1, 4.

———. 1997c. At a Western Outpost of Russia, AIDS Spreads "Like Forest Fire." *New York Times* (4 November): A1, A10.

———. 1998. Citadel of Russia's Wasteful Health System. *New York Times* (4 January): A1, A7.

Stack, Steven, and Elena Bankowski. 1994. Divorce and Drinking: An Analysis of Russian Data. *Journal of Marriage and the Family* 56:805-12.

State Committee of the Russian Federation on Statistics. 1994. *Family in the Russian Federation*. Moscow.

———. 1996. *The Demographic Yearbook of Russia*. Moscow.

Statistisches Bundesamt [Statistical office of the German government]. 1995. *Statistisches Jahrbuch* [Statistical yearbook]. Stuttgart: Metzler and Pöschel.

Stokes, Gale. 1993. *The Walls Came Tumbling Down: The Collapse of Communism in Eastern Europe*. New York: Oxford University Press.

Suny, Ronald Grigor. 1998. *The Soviet Experiment: Russia, the U.S.S.R., and the Successor States*. New York: Oxford University Press.

Sweat, Michael D. and Julie A. Denison. 1995. Reducing HIV Incidence in Developing Countries with Structural and Environmental Interventions. *AIDS* 9:5251–57.

Szadkowska-Stanczyk, J., and W. Hanke. 1991. *Analiza przyczyn wysokiej umieralnosci mezczyzn w wieku w Polsce. Epidemiologiczna ocena ryzyka zgonu z powodu chorob ukladukrazenia* [Causes of high mortality of men at productive age in Poland. Epidemiological evaluation of risks related to cardiovascular deaths]. Warsaw: University of Warsaw School of Economics.

Szantova, M., V. Kupcova, V. Bada, and E. Goncalvesova. 1997. Vyeoj spotreby alkoholu vo vztahu k ochoreniam pecene na Slovensku v rokoch 1973–1994 [Trends in alcohol consumption in relation to liver diseases in Slovakia 1973–1994]. *Bratislavske Lekarske Listy* 98: 12–16.

Szelényi, Ivan, Katherine Beckett, and Lawrence P. King. 1994. The Socialist Economic System. Pp. 234–51 in *Handbook of Economic Sociology*, edited by N. Smelser and R. Swedberg. Princeton, N.J. and New York: Princeton University Press and Russell Sage Foundation.

Sztompka, Piotr. 1993. *The Sociology of Social Change*. Oxford, U.K.: Blackwell.

Tchachenko, G. B., and V. K. Riazantsev. 1993. *Description of the Situation in the Russian Federation*. Copenhagen: WHO Europe Regional Office.

Therborn, Göran. 1995. *European Modernity and Beyond: The Trajectory of European Societies 1945–2000*. London: Sage.

Thiel, C., and L. Heinemann. 1996. Nutritional Behavior Differences in Germany. *Reviews on Environmental Health* 11:35–40.

Thoits, Peggy A. 1995. Stress, Coping, and Social Support Processes: Where Are We? What Next? *Journal of Health and Social Behavior* extra issue:53–79.

Tian-Shanskaia, Olga Semyonova. 1993. *Village Life in Late Tsarist Russia*. Edited by D. Ransel, translated by D. Ransel and M. Levine. Bloomington, Ind.: Indiana University Press.

Tulchinsky, Theodore H., and Elena A. Varavikova. 1996. Addressing the Epidemiologic Transition in the Former Soviet Union: Strategies for Health System and Public Health Reform in Russia. *American Journal of Public Health*. 86:313–20.

Turner, Bryan S. 1988. *Status*. Milton Keynes, U.K.: Open University Press.

———, ed. 1990. *Theories of Modernity and Postmodernity*. London: Sage.

———. 1992. *Regulating Bodies*. London: Routledge.

Turner, R. Jay, Blair Wheaton, and Donald A. Lloyd. 1995. The Epidemiology of Social Stress. *American Sociological Review* 60:125–40.

Uitenbroek, Daan G., Albena Kerekovska, and Nevyana Feschieva. 1996. Health Lifestyle Behavior and Socio-Demographic Characteristics: A Study of Varna, Glasgow, and Edinburgh. *Social Science and Medicine* 43:367–77.

U.S. National Center for Health Statistics. 1997. *Health United States 1996–97.* Washington, D.C.: U.S. Government Printing Office.

Vâlceanu, Daniela. 1992. Inequities in the Health Care System in Romania. Paper presented to the European Society for Health and Medical Sociology meeting, Vienna, September.

Varvasovsky, Zsuzsa, Chris Bain, and Martin McKee. 1996. Deaths from Cirrhosis in Poland and Hungary: The Impact of Different Alcohol Policies During the 1980s. *Journal of Epidemiology and Community Health* 51:167–71.

Volpp, Kevin. 1991. The Structure of Health Care Delivery in Communist East Germany. *Mensch Medizin Gesellschaft* 16:3–13.

Wacquant, Loïc J. D. 1992. Toward a Social Praxeology: The Structure and Logic of Bourdieu's Sociology. Pp. 1-59 in *An Invitation to Reflexive Sociology* by P. Bourdieu and L. Wacquant. Chicago: University of Chicago Press.

Waitzkin, Howard. 1983. *The Second Sickness: Contradictions of Capitalist Health Care.* New York: Free Press.

———. 1989. A Critical Theory of Medical Discourse: Ideology, Social Control, and the Processing of Social Context in Medical Encounters. *Journal of Health and Social Behavior* 30:220–39.

Walters, E. Garrison. 1988. *The Other Europe: Eastern Europe to 1945.* Syracuse, N.Y.: Syracuse University Press.

Watson, Peggy. 1995. Explaining Rising Mortality Among Men in Eastern Europe. *Social Science and Medicine* 41:923–34.

———. 1998. Health Differences in Eastern Europe: Preliminary Findings from the Nowa Huta Study. *Social Science and Medicine* 46:549–58.

Weber, Max. 1946. *From Max Weber: Essays in Sociology.* Edited and translated by H. Gerth and C. Mills. New York: Free Press.

———. 1949. *The Methodology of the Social Sciences.* Translated and edited by E. Shils and H. Finch. New York: Free Press.

———. 1958. *The Protestant Ethic and the Spirit of Capitalism.* New York: Scribners.

———. [1922] 1978. *Economy and Society.* 2 vols. Edited and translated by G. Roth and C. Wittch. Berkeley, Calif.: University of California Press.

Weitz, Eric. 1996. The Heroic Man and the Ever-Changing Woman: Gender and Politics in European Communism, 1917–1950. Pp. 311–52 in *Gender and Class in Modern Europe,* edited by L. Frader and J. Rose. Ithaca, N.Y.: Cornell University Press.

Wilkinson, Richard G. 1996. *Unhealthy Societies: The Afflictions of Inequality.* London: Routledge.

Williams, Simon J. 1995. Theorizing Class, Health and Lifestyles: Can Bourdieu

Help Us? *Sociology of Health and Illness* 17:577–604.

Wnuk-Lipinski, Edmund. 1990. The Polish Country Profile: Economic Crisis and Inequalities in Health. *Social Science and Medicine* 31:859–66.

Wnuk-Lipinski, Edmund, and Raymond Illsley. 1990. International Comparative Analysis: Main Findings and Conclusion. *Social Science and Medicine* 31:879–89.

Wolchik, Sharon L. 1995. The Politics of Transition and the Breakup of Czechoslovakia. Pp. 225–44 in *The End of Czechoslovakia*, edited by J. Musil. Budapest: Central European University Press.

Wong, Raymond Sin-Kwok. 1995. Socialist Stratification and Mobility: Cross-National and Gender Differences in Czechoslovakia, Hungary, and Poland. *Social Science Research* 24:302–28.

World Bank. 1992. *Poland: Health System Reform*. Washington, D.C.: World Bank.

World Health Organization (WHO). 1996. *Health Care Systems in Transition: Romania*. Copenhagen: Regional Office for Europe.

Zágorski, Krzysztof. 1978. The Transformation of Social Structure and Social Mobility in Poland. Pp. 61–80 in *Class Structure & Social Mobility in Poland*, edited by K. Slomczyński and T. Krauze. White Plains, N.Y.: Sharpe.

Zàk, Václav. 1995. The Velvet Divorce—Institutional Foundations. Pp. 245–68 in *The End of Czechoslovakia*, edited by J. Musil. Budapest: Central European University Press.

Zaslavsky, Victor. 1995. From Redistribution to Marketization: Social and Attitudinal Change in Post-Soviet Russia. Pp. 115–142 in *The New Russia: Troubled Transformation*, edited by G. Lapidus. Boulder, Colo.: Westview Press.

Zatonskli, W., A. McMichael, and A. Powles. 1998. Ecological Study of Reasons for Sharp Decline in Mortality from Ischaemic Heart Disease in Poland since 1991. *British Medical Journal* 316:1047–51.

Zotov, V. D. 1985. *The Marxist-Leninist Theory of Society*. Moscow: Progress Publishers.

Zubeck, Voytek. 1990. Walesa's Leadership and Poland's Tradition. *Problems of Communism* XL:69–83.

———. 1993. The Fragmentation of Poland's Political Party System. *Communist and Post-Communist Studies* 26:47–71.

———. 1997. The Eclipse of Walesa's Political Career. *Europe-Asia Studies* 49:107–24.

Subject Index

Author Index